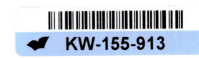

DIRECTIONS
a guide to **Key Documents**
in **Health and Social Care**
2004

4th edition
edited by: Lyn Crecy

Contributors:

Anne Brown
Lyn Crecy
Anne Henderson
Susan Martin
Nicola Tricker

University of Plymouth

London: TSO

Published by TSO (The Stationery Office) and available from:

Online
www.tso.co.uk/bookshop

Mail, Telephone, Fax & E-mail
TSO
PO Box 29, Norwich, NR3 1GN
Telephone orders/General enquiries: 0870 600 5522
Fax orders: 0870 600 5533
E-mail: book.orders@tso.co.uk
Textphone: 0870 240 3701

TSO Shops
123 Kingsway, London, WC2B 6PQ
020 7242 6393 Fax 020 7242 6394
68-69 Bull Street, Birmingham B4 6AD
0121 236 9696 Fax 0121 236 9699
9-21 Princess Street, Manchester M60 8AS
0161 834 7201 Fax 0161 833 0634
16 Arthur Street, Belfast BT1 4GD
028 9023 8451 Fax 028 9023 5401
18-19 High Street, Cardiff CF10 1PT
029 2039 5548 Fax 029 2038 4347
71 Lothian Road, Edinburgh EH3 9AZ
0870 606 5566 Fax 0870 606 5588

TSO Accredited Agents
(see Yellow Pages)

and through good booksellers

This is the fourth edition of
A guide to key documents in health care for nurses, midwives and health visitors 1986-1997
Originally published in 1997

Fourth edition 2005

ISBN 0 11 703476 2

for editorial enquiries contact:
Lyn Crecy
Subject Librarian: Health Studies, University of Plymouth
Learning Resources Service, Somerset College of Arts and Technology,
Wellington Road, TAUNTON TA1 5AX Somerset
tel: 01823 366454
fax: 01823 366411
email: lcrecy@plymouth.ac.uk

Printed in the United Kingdom for The Stationery Office
174932 C15 02/05

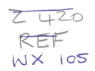

DIRECTIONS
a guide to **Key Documents** in Health and Social Care
2004

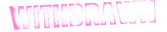

Contents

Introduction

This is the fourth edition of a guide to more than 200 key reports and legislation published on health and social care in over eighteen years.

It offers:
- a guide for students embarking on health, medical and social care careers
- a reminder of the main landmarks for those going to interview
- a background of information for individuals new to health and social care

The new edition has been expanded to include a new chapter: **Ethical Issues & Human Rights**. All other sections have been revised and updated. Documents should be available to borrow or request from your local academic or medical library; many are available in full text on the internet. *Directions* is divided into 11 chapters arranged as follows:

1. General
2. Quality
3. Public Health
4. Primary Care
5. Older People
6. Midwifery
7. Children and Young People
8. Mental Health
9. Disabilities
10. Education
11. Ethical Issues and Human Rights

The headings are very broad and not mutually exclusive. The documents are arranged in chronological order and each is referenced with an abstract. Where there has been discussion in the press, this has been added as further reading. Many of the documents stem one from another and so we created a **chronological index** at the front, with page references.

For those who will be using the guide to prepare for job interviews, **Applying for Jobs** contains some helpful reading. *Directions* also lists the main **national organisations** that influence health and social care, gives their contact details and a brief statement of purpose. There are short lists of **abbreviations** and **websites**, and finally an **alphabetical index** at the back.

The range of documents is not exhaustive: (at times, documents are specific to England only, for example) but it includes those that have been 'most asked for' in our experience; where appropriate, chapters include a list of **supplementary reading**. As new policies and reports emerge, *Directions* will be updated. In the meantime, any ideas or amendments are welcome.

The abstracts are the authors' own, resulting from reading the original documents. They are meant to offer a broad outline of policy and thinking in health and social care but in no way do they replace the originals. If you need to read *NHS plan (2000)* you must read it, the author accepts no responsibility for any misunderstandings or decisions made on the basis of the text of this book.

For their help in the production of this guide, I should like to thank my colleagues, in the FHSW and ILS at the University of Plymouth as well as Richard Middleton at the Editorial Offices of The Stationery Office.

Lyn Crecy, Learning Resources Service,
Somerset College, Wellington Road, TAUNTON TA1 5AX

December 2004

Chronological Index

1 General

Department of Health (1989) *Working for patients: the health service: caring for the 1990s (cm 555).* London: HMSO

Summary: a white paper that proposes seven key measures with the aim of giving patients greater choice and of increasing efficiency. The seven measures would implement reforms in the following areas:

- responsibility at local level
- self-governing trusts
- purchasers/providers being able to offer and receive services in other health authorities, with funding crossing administrative boundaries
- an increase consultant posts to reduce waiting times
- GP fundholding
- a streamlining of management structure based on regions introducing executive and non-executive directors
- to introduce medical audit to ensure quality of services is maintained

The document followed the Conservative Government's review of the NHS and introduced the most radical reforms in the NHS since its foundation in 1948.

Further reading:
Horne, E. M. (1989) Working for patients: begging the questions?....future management of the NHS. *Professional Nurse* 4(7) 318
Wheeler, N. (1990) "Working for patients" and "Caring for people" the same philosophy? *British Journal of Occupational Therapy* 53(10) 409-14

Department of Health (1990) *The National Health Service and Community Care Act 1990: chapter 19.* London: HMSO

Summary: the first legislative reform of the NHS since its founding in 1948. Arises from the two white papers: *Working for patients (1989)* and *Caring for people (1991).*

Makes five key points:

1. QUALITY: as the result of the introduction of market forces, there should be explicit standards of care and patient information (Patient's charter 1991); measurable outcomes and evidence-based practice.
2. FLEXIBILITY: this legislates for the concept of a NEEDS-led service instead of the other way around. Health services to be redeveloped to suit needs of individuals, communities and populations.

3. CHOICE: purchasers of health services - e.g. GP fundholders - free to choose from a range of providers.

4. ACCOUNTABILITY: to establish who is responsible for delivering what health care: the responsibilities of the various care-giving agencies to be properly defined.

5. PARTNERSHIP: this is to legislate for good cooperation between: hospital and community agencies, statutory, voluntary and independent organisations, and between patients, professionals and informal carers.

Council of the European Union (1993) *European working time directive no. 93/104/EC.* Brussels: Council of the European Union

Summary: a directive to limit the working hours of all European workers to:

*   58 hours per week by August 2004, to 56 hours by 2007 and to 48 hours by August 2009. This was particularly significant for NHS junior doctors who regularly worked 72 hour weeks including on-call time

*   also provides for 11 hours continuous rest in every 24; 24 hours continuous rest in every 7 days; 20 minute breaks in work periods over six hours; night work not exceeding eight hours in every 24 and four weeks annual leave

*   whilst giving due consideration to workers' health and safety, member states may elect to "opt out" because of special circumstances

These provisions were modified by the following court cases:

*   the SIMAP Judgement (2000): following an claim by Spanish doctors, the European Court of Justice ruled that on-call time, spent at one's place of work, **should** be considered part of the 48-hour working week. However, where doctors were on-call but not at their place of work, this was **not** to be considered 'working time'

*   the Jaegar Judgement (2003): a German Dr Jaeger claimed that time 'on-call' in hospital was essentially working time, whereas his employers insisted that time spent on-call but not working should be treated as 'rest time'. The Court ruled that unlike doctors on standby who were **not** "on the premises", on-call working "on the premises" **should** be regarded as working time even where there were facilities for rest and sleep

Further reading:

Exten-Wright, J. (1997) Europe's working time directive: how it will affect junior doctors. *British Journal of Health Care Management* 3(9) 495-6

Exten-Wright, J. and Hannon, J. (2001) Working time directive: legal implications. *British Journal of Health Care Management* 7(3) 102-3

Finch, J. (1997) Trainee doctors in the UK, and the EC working time directive: a note on stress and working time. *European Journal of Health Law* 4(1) 69-79

NHS Executive (1998) *Working time directive agreement for career grade doctors.* London: Department of Health

Greenhalgh & Co. (1994) *The interface between junior doctors and nurses: a research study for the Department of Health.* (chair Kenneth Calman) Macclesfield: Greenhalgh & Co.

Summary: the aim of the research was "to contribute to the improvement in patient care by examining the interface between junior hospital doctors and ward nurses, with a view to enhancing the role of nurses and reducing the inappropriate role of junior hospital doctors."

The researchers looked at three areas:

- what junior doctors do
- what work is transferable between junior doctors and nurses for the benefit of patients
- areas of good practice

The report recommends six activities that nurses should undertake emphasising that these "should be shared with junior doctors not merely transferred to nurses". These activities should be part of the role of all registered nurses and do not need to be undertaken by specialists or nurse practitioners.

These activities are:

- taking a patient history
- venous blood sampling
- insertion of a peripheral IV cannula
- referring a patient for an investigation
- writing discharge letters to GPs and other doctors
- administration of drugs (excluding cytotoxic and first doses) via peripheral IV cannula

The report suggests that joint planning of care and collaborative practice between junior doctors and nurses should be pursued. Joint education for practice and competency testing in the activities identified should be included in the core curriculum for pre-registration nursing and undergraduate medical training.

Further reading:
Richardson, G. and Maynard, A. (1995) *Fewer doctors? More nurses? A review of the knowledge base of doctor-nurse substitution.* York: University of York

Audit Commission (1995) *The doctors' tale: the work of hospital doctors in England and Wales.* London: Audit Commission

Summary: the report presents a picture of doctors under increasing pressure owing to advances in technology, greater patient expectations and the need for efficiency. On the other hand doctors' work is often poorly defined, consultants' commitments are not clear, there is an uneven skill mix and workloads vary enormously, often to the detriment of personal and family lives. Medical training is poorly organised and inflexible with insufficient supervision for junior doctors, many with no named supervisor.

Recommendations include:

- clinical directors to take a lead role in managing doctors of all grades
- doctors' responsibilities to be made explicit, with "job" plans completed for all consultants and consideration given to work that could be passed to nurses or other staff
- service and training needs should be clearer and more structured: royal colleges to set standards of competence for trainees and trusts to write policies for doctors' professional development
- working practices should be more efficient with greater use of shifts in order to reduce the working hours of junior doctors and to allow for doctors who have family commitments

Further reading:
Butler, P. (1995) A sting in the tale. *Health Service Journal* 105(5444) 11

Sims, J. (1995) Will job plans stop the spying? *Healthcare Management* 3(4) 16-8

Department of Health (1996) *The National Health Service: a service with ambitions (cm 3425).* London: The Stationery Office

Summary: the Government outlines the fundamental principles on which the NHS was founded and restates its continued commitment to them. To these principles is added the requirement for a responsive and sensitive service in which the needs of the individual are met. Through a series of case studies, the Government demonstrates the kind of care that people should expect if the government's ambitions are to be realised. This will come about by setting five strategic objectives namely: a well-informed public, a seamless service, knowledge-based decision-making, a highly trained and skilled workforce and a responsive service.

The paper states that future pressures on the NHS such as medical advances, population changes and public expectations are manageable: the NHS has adapted and continues to adapt to change. Finally, the paper details several specific areas which need to be addressed. These are in the area of primary care (see Chapter 2), professional development and the provision of information.

Further reading:
News focus. (1996) *Health Service Journal* 106(5528) 12-13

Department of Health (1997) *The new NHS: modern, dependable (cm3807).* London: The Stationery Office

Summary: white paper stressing the importance of primary care. The government proposes substantial savings (£1 billion) on administrative costs, to be transferred directly to patient care, by replacing the internal market with "integrated care". This is to be achieved by the following initiatives:

- quality and efficiency to be improved and monitored by a National Institute for Clinical Excellence, setting evidence-based guidelines for clinicians. Some issues raised here are developed in *A first class service (1998)*

- introduction of Primary Care Groups (PCGs) made up of GPs and community nurses, to commission services from NHS Trusts on a long-term rather than annual basis. These PCGs replace fundholder groups
- fewer health authorities covering larger areas

The separation of planning and provision of care will continue.

Major developments in direct services to patients are:

1. NHS Direct, a 24-hour telephone advice service staffed by nurses, to be implemented nationally by 2000
2. all GPs connected to NHS Net by 2002 to speed up both booking of outpatient appointments and patients' results
3. improved cancer services with specialist appointments within 2 weeks of referral, to be implemented by 2000

Further reading:

Crail, M. (1997) Modern times. *Health Service Journal* 107(5583) 10-11

Crofts, L. (1998) Good news down the line. *Nursing Times* 94(28) 34-36

Keighley T (1998) Yvonne Moores. *Nursing Management* 4(10) 17-20

News: the NHS white paper (1997) *Nursing Standard* 12 (13/15) 36-37

NHS Executive (1998) *A consultation on a strategy for nursing, midwifery and health visiting (HSC 1998/045).* London: Department of Health

Payne, D. (1997) Primary movers. *Nursing Times* 95(51) 8-9

J. M. Consulting (1998) *The regulation of nurses, midwives and health visitors: report on a review of the Nurses, Midwives and Health Visitors Act 1997.* Bristol: J.M. Consulting Ltd

Summary: as an independent consultancy, J.M. Consulting were commissioned by the Department of Health to review the most recent legislation governing the profession. The review was achieved by extensive consultation with the statutory bodies (UKCC and the four national boards) and with individuals, focus groups and representatives from nurse education providers. The main areas of concern are:

- protecting patients from unsafe practices
- new training arrangements and nurses' changing role
- accountability
- political devolution in the UK

The report identifies weaknesses and omissions in the legislation and recommends a new Act to regulate the professions with following recommendations:

- a new, single body to replace the UKCC and 4 national boards
- to improve standards, parity of representation for both nursing and midwifery
- the inclusion of lay advisors to assist the work of the new body
- a revised code of conduct
- the abolition of separate registration for health visitors
- the four UK health departments to regulate the training and practice of health care support workers

In February 1999, the Government publicly endorsed the review's recommendations but maintain that health visitors should continue to have separate registration.

Further reading:

Chaffer, D. (1998) Learn about plans for the health service tomorrow. *Nursing Standard* 12(24 No Limits supplement) 49

Downe, S. (1998) Legislation and professional autonomy: is there a conflict? *British Journal of Midwifery* 6(4) 234

Keighley, T. (1998) Structuring health care for the future. *Nursing Management* 5(3) 23-7

Lewis, Paul (1999) Review of the Nurses, Midwives and Health Visitors Act. *British Journal of Midwifery* 7(4) 214-5

Audit Commission (1999) *Cover story: the use of locum doctors in NHS trusts.* London: Audit Commission

Summary: on a typical day, 3,500 locums are employed to cover job vacancies, annual and sick leave at a cost of £214 million per annum. This can lead to problems of care because:

- with short postings (often less than two days), the locum may have only a poor induction to the setting and its procedures
- some locums have not held a permanent post for some time and their education and training may not be up-to-date
- pre-employment checks are not thorough

This can lead to unnecessary expense because agencies pay more per hour and trusts' systems for employing locums are inconsistent and poorly managed. Systems are open to fraud. Recommendations include:

- an accreditation system to ensure locums are working to a high standard
- all locums to be assured of an individual performance review
- trusts to appoint a senior doctor to lead and be accountable for all doctors employed in this way
- for better value for money, trusts to set up contracts with agencies

The Health Act 1999: chapter 8. London: The Stationery Office

Summary: principally a reform of primary care, replacing GP fundholding with primary care trusts.

- outlines the functions of primary care trusts and their mechanisms for funding and expenditure
- primary care and NHS trusts to establish a "duty of quality" to monitor and improve the quality of health care
- a Commission for Health Improvement (CHI) will provide advice and information to trusts about meeting their duty of quality
- the CHI will have the power to carry out reviews and investigations into the management, availability and quality of care and (subject to regulation) may

inspect premises, inspect and take copies of any documentation and publish without consent if there is considered to be risk to the welfare of patients. Subject to regulation the CHI may also charge the bodies responsible for the cost of the CHI's investigation

- Health Authorities and Trusts must work collaboratively
- Health Authorities to draw up Health Improvement Programmes; Local Authorities and NHS trusts to cooperate.

The Act gives the Health Secretary the power to curb drug prices. It also legislates to modernise professional self-regulation: by-passing the customary parliamentary debate, the Health Secretary has the power to alter professional regulation.

Further reading:
Whitfield, L. (1999) After Henry. *Health Service Journal* 109(5641) 10-11

UKCC (1999) *A higher level of practice.* London: UKCC

Summary: discusses proposals for setting and regulating a generic standard for a higher level of practice with a system for assessment and a charge levied for the assessment process.

Department of Health (1999) *Making a difference: strengthening the nursing, midwifery and health visiting contribution to health and health care.* London: Department of Health

Summary: aims to increase the contribution that nurses, midwives and health visitors make to health care by maximising their potential. Chapters include:

- recruitment: improving and expanding the workforce, and increasing student places
- education: more flexible training with longer and enhanced practical placements. A *Partners Council* to oversee post-qualifying education and development
- careers: a modernised pay system is planned with three ranges for registered staff and a fourth for cadets and health care assistants. Progression will be linked to responsibilities and competencies; new consultant posts will extend career and pay opportunities
- improving working lives: practitioners to be involved in decision-making. Employers must offer family-friendly work arrangements and must protect staff by tackling discrimination, accidents, violence and harassment
- quality: practitioners to contribute to the National Service Frameworks, clinical governance and evidence-based practice
- leadership: practitioners to be supported to develop leadership and management skills
- self-regulations: must be open, responsive and accountable; Government to establish new regulatory framework
- extended role: the Government supports prescribing, nurse/midwife – led services and the potential for practitioners to increase their responsibilities

Further reading:
Hancock, C. (1999) Perspectives. *Nursing Standard* 13(43) 22

Strategy for nursing. *Nursing Standard* 13(43) 4-5

Department of Health (1999) *Review of prescribing, supply and administration of medicines: final report.* (chair June Crown) London: Department of Health

Summary: after outlining the present situation of who may prescribe, supply and administer drugs, the report proposes extending prescribing powers and setting criteria for approving, training and regulating new prescribers. Defines two kinds of prescribers. The "independent" prescriber has the first contact with the patient and is responsible for the initial assessment, diagnosis and prescription. The "dependent" prescriber is responsible for the continuing care of the patient and may vary the frequency and dose of the original prescription. Good communication between the two parties is essential and to be regulated. The prime motivation of the report is improved patient care and an increase of patient choice.

Further reading:
Department of Health (1989) *Report of the advisory group on nurse prescribing.* London: Department of Health

Karen Luker et al (1997) *Evaluation of nurse prescribing: final report.* Liverpool: The University of Liverpool

Edwards, M. (1999) The Crown report: a new prescribing framework. *British Journal of Community Health Nursing* 4(5) 212

Department of Health (2000) *Comprehensive critical care: a review of adult critical care services.* London: Department of Health

Summary: a three-five year modernisation programme. Proposals are made for every sector involved in critical care with examples of good practice. The existing division into high dependency and intensive care to be replaced by a classification that identifies four levels of care and can identify specialties such as renal, thoracic, surgical etc.

Critical care services should feature four characteristics:

- integration: there should a hospital-wide approach to critical care with support and communication between all the involved agencies
- networks: several trusts to integrate their services, working to common standards to provide the full range of critical care services within a geographical area
- workforce development: there should a planned approach to all personnel issues including education and training and involving all levels of staff
- data collecting culture promoting an evidence base: effective information gathering promotes good patient outcomes and turns a reactive service into a proactive one

Further reading:
Audit Commission (1999) *Critical to success: the place of efficient and effective critical care services within the acute hospital.* London: Audit Commission

Hogan, J. (2000) Staff ratios in intensive care: are they adequate? *British Journal of Nursing* 9(13) 817

Wright, Mike (2000) Intensive pressure. *Nursing Times* 96(33) 29-30

Meadows, S. Levenson, Ros and Baeza, Juan (2000) *The last straw: explaining the NHS nursing shortage.* London: King's Fund

Summary: the result of a literature review and a series of interviews and focus groups with NHS nurses and managers. Nurses are leaving the NHS faster than they are being recruited: of a total workforce of 330,000, the shortfall is estimated to be between 8,000 and 13,000.

Reasons given:

- low pay
- bleak working conditions
- lack of control
- discrimination and harassment of black and ethnic minority workers

The authors recommend:

- managers to listen to nurses
- ensuring career development for all
- eliminating discrimination
- offering support and flexible working hours

Further reading:
Audit Commission (1997) *Finders keepers: the management of staff turnover in NHS trusts.* London: Audit Commission

Carvel, John (2001) NHS recruitment: search for staff to fulfil health pledges. *The Guardian* 23.5.01

Davies, J. (2000) Finders, keepers. *Health Service Journal* 110(5733) 24-9

NHS Executive (2000) *Meeting the challenge: a strategy for allied health professions.* London: Department of Health

Summary: a strategy designed to bring allied health professionals (such as podiatrists, radiographers, speech therapists etc) into line with the rest of health and social care services as part of the *NHS plan: a plan for investment, a plan for reform (2000).* The strategy allows a four-year timescale and includes the following proposals:

- changes to be overseen by an Allied Health Professions forum
- workforce to expand from 50,000 to 60,000 and to include new Consultant Therapist posts by 2004
- services to be made faster and more accessible
- improve care for in heart disease, cancer and mental illnesses and for older people
- care to be patient-focused and protocol-based
- improve interagency communication within health and social care services
- professions to be regulated by a Health Professions Council with a single register

Department of Health (2000) *The NHS plan: a plan for investment; a plan for reform (cm4818-I).* London: The Stationery Office

Summary: a ten-year plan promising financial investment for:

- personnel - 7,500 more consultants, 2,000 more GPs, 20,000 more nurses
- beds - 7,000 more by 2004
- cleaner hospitals - 'clean up' campaign to start immediately
- equipment for cancer, kidney and heart disease services
- a National Performance Fund
- twenty diagnostic and and treatment centres for day and short stay surgery
- hospitals - 100 new hospitals by 2010 as well as 500 primary care centres

The reforms include:

- contracts that commit consultants to working up to seven years for the NHS with reward for further commitment
- faster access: by 2005, waiting times for operations to be reduced to six months and outpatient appointments to three months. Where an operation is cancelled for non-clinical reasons, patient to be funded for a private operation
- nurses to gain greater prescribing powers as well as the power to admit and discharge patients
- a new level of Primary Care Trusts to commission total health and social care packages
- Community Health Councils to be replaced by patient advocacy services and patient forums
- a national framework for working in the private sector
- the appointment of senior sisters ('modern matrons') in hospitals to control resources in order to improve standards of care. They will have the authority to intervene to sort out discharge delays and poor hygiene
- nurse consultant posts increased to 1000
- special improvements in services for care of patients with heart disease, cancer and mental illness as well as elderly people

Further reading:

Anon (2000) The national plan for the NHS: your essential guide. *Nursing Times* 96 (31) 4-7

Calman, K. et al (2002) *Make or break time? A commentary on Labour's health policy two years into the NHS plan.* Durham: University of Durham

Castledine, George (2000) Reinforcing the medical stereotypes of nursing. *British Journal of Nursing* 9(15) 1026

Hunter, D. J. (2001) The NHS plan: a new direction for English public health? *Critical Public Health* 11(1) 75-81

Commission on the National Health Service (2000) *New life for health.* (chair Will Hutton) London: Vintage

Summary: this report was commissioned by the Association of Community Health Councils for England and Wales and is the result of a study of the NHS including a telephone poll of the public conducted in March 2000.

The poll:

- 63% believed the NHS was our most valuable institution
- 60% felt the NHS needed improvement
- 96% believed that free medical treatment at the time of need - the basic tenet of the NHS since its inception - should be a basic British right

The Commission found that by any standards, service delivery in the NHS is very low and that there is a growing gap between delivery and expectation. The 3 main reasons for this are:

1. low finance has meant that some services such as dentistry and long-term care are not always available on the NHS
2. the internal market led to inequality of care, although the establishment of NICE and the CHI has gone some way to remedy this
3. an absence of accountability and 'transparent' decision-making: there is no solid 'settled' system of patient rights, the NHS bill for medical negligence currently stands at £3 billion, overall the NHS ethos is defensive and based on blame

The Commission makes two radical recommendations:

1. the Government to consult the public in writing a constitution for the NHS that would represent shared principles irrespective of party politics
2. the NHS to become a national institution similar to the BBC or the Bank of England: independent of government control but with Government having overall "arm's length" responsibility

Further reading:
Watt, N. (2000) Ministers should let go control of the NHS. *The Guardian* 18.4.00
Miles, Alice (2000) Patients do not have a cure for the NHS. *The Times* 25.4.00

Department of Health (2000) *Shaping the future NHS: long term planning for hospitals and related services: consultation document on the findings of the National Beds Inquiry.* London: The Stationery Office

Summary: the National Beds Inquiry was set up to look at the hospital beds situation ten to twenty years ahead. Concerns about the pressures on emergency beds during the winter and the length of hospital waiting lists led to the establishment of the Inquiry. It has three aims:

- to investigate the key resources needed by the NHS in the long term, and to assess the future impact of current policies and other factors, taking into account the wider picture

- to consult with the NHS and partner agencies about these investigations and involve them in discussions about developments (especially about hospital beds) over the next 10 to 20 years
- to assist with long-term planning by producing a common set of assumptions from their findings

Health and Social Care Act 2001: chapter 15. London: The Stationery Office

Summary: intended to support the policies set out in the NHS plan (2000) and the Government's response to the Royal Commission on long term care (2000):

- provides for funding the NHS and family health services, including payments for new initiatives and intervention for those organisations with poor performance
- provides for piloting community pharmacy services including 'by remote means' such as via the internet or by mail order
- provides for the establishment of Care Trusts
- provides for the funding for long-term care; excludes nursing care and makes local authorities responsible for care arrangements
- provides for the Secretary of State to permit the sharing of confidential information if it is in the interests of patient care or public welfare
- extends prescribing power to certain nurses, midwives and health visitors

Audit Commission (2001) *Brief encounters: getting the best from temporary nursing staff.* London: Audit Commission

Summary: on any single day, 20,000 bank or agency nurses are employed to cover sick leave, job vacancies, annual leave and to a much lesser extent, study and maternity leave. This can lead to poor quality care because nurses are assigned to unfamiliar settings, inductions and handovers are rarely given and pre-employment checks are not thoroughly carried out (e.g. work permits, UKCC registration, occupational health checks and police records). The situation presents poor value for money because time is wasted due to poor planning, agencies commonly pay 20-25% more than nursing banks and the systems for filling in timesheets and claims forms are open to fraud and exploitation. Recommendations include:

- to ensure pre-employment checks are made and inductions properly given
- to ensure all temporary staff receive basic training, especially in emergency procedures, lifting and handling etc and to support bank staff's applications for training
- to ensure proper control of timesheets and payment claims
- trusts to open contracts with agencies
- to ensure more cost effective and less reactive staff planning, with central coordination of staff cover and standardised processes that make better use of information technology

Further reading:
Mahony, Chris et al (2001) Watchdog's verdict: millions squandered, nurses neglected: Nursing Times special feature. *Nursing Times* 97(36) 10-13

NHS Executive (2001) *Making the change: a strategy for the professions in healthcare science.* London: Department of Health

Summary: a four-year plan designed to raise standards on the one hand and on the other, raise the public profile and working conditions of health care scientists. The different professions included in health care science are described and the plan's proposals include:

- the development of a National Occupational Standards Framework in healthcare science to define best practice and direct education and training
- to replace the Council for Professions Supplementary to Medicine with a new Health Professions Council and a single Health Professions Register
- enhance public confidence by raising healthcare scientists' profiles
- modernise education and training and improve healthcare science career opportunities in order to raise standards and resolve problems with recruitment and retention

Department of Health (2001) *Shifting the balance of power within the NHS: securing delivery.* London: Department of Health

Summary: as an extension of the *NHS plan (2000)* this consultation paper plans for the reform of management by shifting emphasis to 'frontline' staff working in the community. The four main points are:

1. Primary Care Trusts (PCTs) to become the lead organisation in assessing, planning and commissioning health services and to work at new partnerships with local agencies and local government. Resources to be allocated directly to the Trusts rather than via Health Authorities
2. NHS Trusts to continue to provide services whilst devolving responsibility to clinical teams and promoting clinical networks across the NHS. High performance to be rewarded
3. the 95 local Health Authorities to be replaced by 30 Strategic Health Authorities that will look at the strategic development of health services as well as performance and accountability of the Trusts
4. Department of Health Regional Offices to be replaced by four Directors of Health and Social Care, overseers who will provide the link between the NHS and the Department of Health. NHS staff and services to be supported by three new bodies: The Modernisation Agency, the Leadership Centre and the University of the NHS

The *NHS Reform and Health Care Professions Act 2002* legislates for the changes.

Further reading:

Bamford, Terry et al (2001) Thoughts on shifting the balance of power. *British Journal of Health Care Management* 7(9) 355-7

Dixon, M. (2002) Shifting the balance of power: managing change. *British Journal of Health Care Management* 8(3) 104-7

Graham, Alison and Steele, Jane (2001) *Optimising value.* London: Public Management Foundation

Walshe, Kieran and Smith, Judith (2001) Cause and effect. *Health Service Journal* 111(5776) 20-3

Department of Health (2001) *Implementing the NHS plan: modern matrons: strengthening the role of ward sisters and introducing senior sisters: HSC2001/10.* London: Department of Health

Summary: proposes a new role for senior sisters and charge nurses: Matrons to be responsible for a group of wards and act as a clear authority and trouble shooter for patients and families as well as a clinical authority for working nurses. Matrons will have the power and budget to sort out fundamentals of care, in particular:

- cleanliness
- enhancing the ward environment with support from new Ward Housekeepers and ward environment budgets
- hospital food
- essence of care benchmarks
- hospital acquired infection
- taking a lead in empowering nurses through developing clinical leadership and the Chief Nursing Officer's Ten key roles for nurses (2003)

Further reading:
Department of Health (2002) *Modern matrons in the NHS: a progress report.* London: Department of Health

Oughtibridge, D. (2003) The modern matron. *Nursing Management* 10(2) 26-8

Snell, J. (2001) Thoroughly modern matron. *Health Service Journal* 111(5744) 28-31

National Health Service Reform and Health Care Professions Act 2002: chapter 17. London: The Stationery Office

Summary: arises from proposals made in *Shifting the balance of power (2001) Involving patients and public in healthcare (2001)* and the *Kennedy report (2001).* The Act provides as follows:

- Health Authorities to be renamed Strategic Health Authorities (SHA) with most of their functions passing to PCTs who will receive funds direct and be responsible for service planning. SHAs to manage the performance of health services provided in their area
- strengthens the power and independence of CHI, making clear that health care inspection must extend to the patient's environment. CHI to inspect and report on NHS services, reporting directly to the Secretary of State where there are serious concerns
- independent 'Patients' forums' to be set up in every trust to represent patients and the public and promote involvement in local decision-making. Patients' Forums in PCTs will commission and provide Independent Advocacy Services
- establish a Commission for Patient and Public Involvement in Health
- Community Health Councils to be abolished
- prison health care to come under the aegis of the NHS

- a Council for the Regulation of Health Care Professionals will oversee the work of regulatory bodies such as the General Medical Council, the NMC and Royal Pharmaceutical Society. This will coordinate good practice and other aspects of their work as well as handle appeal cases concerning fitness to practice

Further reading:
House of Commons Health Committee (2003) *Patient and public involvement in the NHS.* London: The Stationery Office

Finlayson, B. (2002) *Counting the smiles: morale and motivation in the NHS.* London: King's Fund

Summary: the result of a literature review and a series of focus groups with NHS personnel, motivated by NHS plans for modernisation set against the fact that staff are still leaving the service in 'significant' numbers. Three factors that have an impact on morale are:

1. whether staff feel cared for
2. the quality of the working environment: e.g. staff levels and workloads, too many changes and upheavals, no opportunities for staff development
3. pay and resources: low salaries depressed staff less than when there were insufficient funds for the service itself

The report endorses the *Improving working lives standard (2001)* making the following recommendations:

- value staff: through compliments; senior managers taking a genuine interest in frontline work; involving staff in decisions
- employ sufficient numbers
- sustain the investment in staff pay but more especially in the service itself
- recruitment and retention drives needed especially in the inner cities

Wanless, D., Health Trends Review Team and HM Treasury (2002) *Securing our future health: taking a long-term view.* London: HM Treasury

Summary: a report commissioned by the Chancellor of the Exchequer whose interim report revealed how poorly the UK compared with other countries in 'health outcomes' with a history of inadequate and badly managed funding. This report aims to present a vision of the NHS in 2022 with what financial and other resources will be needed to keep the NHS providing a high quality, publicly funded service that is free at the point of need. Wanless views as 'ambitious' the hope that the NHS will 'catch up' in only twenty years. At present the pressure on resources comes from:

- existing commitments
- raised expectation
- advancing technology and drug developments
- changing demography
- inflation
- improvements in productivity

The report offers three viable scenarios with cost estimates for each:

1. Solid Progress - in which there is an increase in life expectancy and public engagement with their health

2. Slow Uptake - no increase in life expectancy or public engagement

3. Fully Engaged - here there are high levels of public engagement, a high increase in life expectancy and a high increase in health status

Continuous, rigorous audit and review are essential to success. The workforce would have to develop in skillmix as well as increase in manpower and social care would have to be fully integrated. The report projects spending to rise from the current £68 billion to between £154 and £184 billion over the 20 years. To achieve the plan on less would need: improvement in productivity, greater success in public health, taking longer than twenty years, letting go of improvements that weren't value for money.

Further reading:

Appleby, J. et al (2004) *How much should we spend on the NHS: issues and challenges arising from the Wanless review of future health care spending.* London: King's Fund

Health Trends Review Team (2002) *Health care systems in eight countries: trends and challenges.* London: London School of Economics and Political Science

Kendall, L. (2002) After Wanless: health outcomes and spending targets. *New Economy* 9(1) 16-20

Department of Health (2002) *Delivering the NHS plan: next steps on investment: next steps on reform (cm5503).* London: The Stationery Office

Summary: Government remains convinced that general taxation is still the best way to ensure no one is left out of care provision, and aims to bring health spending up to 9.4% of the country's GDP by 2008 - on a par with the rest of Europe. Whilst upholding the 1948 principle that care be provided free at the point of need, the model of care has to change, from top-down management to a devolved system that offers diverse, needs-led care bound by common standards and tough inspection. The promised benefits of extra spending include:

- waiting times reduced, e.g. for operations from 15 to 6 months by 2003 and to 3 months by 2008

- employing increased numbers of doctors, therapists, scientists, nurses and midwives

- greater funding available for training staff for the future

- best practice spread through the NSFs and NICE guidance, supported by the NHS Modernisation Agency

What is planned for the future includes:

- stronger incentives to ensure cash is spent on service improvement

- bringing us in line with Europe, hospitals to be paid through a system of "payment by results", i.e. those units that do more will be paid more

- over four years from 2002, introducing Scandinavian system that offers patients a choice of provider. By 2005 appointments will be booked for a time and place convenient to the patient, whether it be at an NHS or private hospital locally or elsewhere, including overseas. The private sector will continue to be used where they can genuinely serve the NHS

- as a measure for devolution, consideration will be given for an 'arms' length' NHS bank, allowing the NHS itself to invest capital and allow for long-term planning
- PCTs to hold 75% of the NHS budget
- hospitals with proven track record may apply for 'foundation' status which will give them greater independence from central government and the freedom to control assets, invest revenue gained from land sales and reward staff
- to improve the relationship with health services especially in elderly care, social services will be given incentives to improve care homes and home care services to older people
- there will be radical change in the job design and pay system (see *Agenda for change, 2004* and *Knowledge and skills framework, 2003*)
- tougher inspection legislation will lead to the appointment of a Chief Inspector of Health Care, reporting to Parliament and the establishment of CHAI - the Commission for Healthcare Audit and Inspection (replaces the Commission for Health Improvement) and CSCI - the Commission for Social Care Inspection

Further Reading:

Cunningham, D. (2002) The NHS plan and clinicians. *Clinical Medicine* 2(2) 134-8

Department of Health (2002) *NHS foundations trusts: eligibility, criteria and timetable.* London: Department of Health

Eyres, J. and Dewar, S. (2002) Constrained innovation and the NHS plan. *British Journal of Health Care Management* 8(3) 101-3

House of Commons Health Committee (2003) *Second report: foundation trusts: HC395-II.* London: The Stationery Office

Newman, K and Maylor, U. (2002) The NHS plan: nurse satisfaction, commitment and retention strategies. *Health Services Management Research* 15(2) 93-105

Department of Health (2002) *Reforming NHS financial flows: introducing payment by results.* London: Department of Health

Summary: a programme of financial reform extending five years from 2003. Principles are:

- financial management should be transparent
- supports offering patients a choice of providers
- high quality and efficiency should be rewarded
- helps match demand to capacity
- system should be driven by the needs of the population

The system involves coding every activity and paying hospitals and trusts for those activities according to a nationally set tariff, with casemix and volume of work established by Healthcare Resources Groups.

Further reading:

Audit Commission (2003) *Introducing payment by results: getting the balance right for the NHS and taxpayers.* London: Audit Commission

Dixon, J. (2004) Payment by results: new financial flows in the NHS. *British Medical Journal* 328(7446) 969-70

Department of Health (2003) *Building on the best: choice, responsiveness and equity in the NHS (cm6079).* London: The Stationery Office

Summary: the result of a consultation exercise involving over 110,000 people. Issues include:

- patients want a share in decision-making based on getting good information at the right time; they want the NHS to listen and respond to their views
- patients want the NHS to adapt to them, instead of having to adapt themselves
- the NHS should continue to grow, with improvements in particular for people with long-term illnesses
- power should continue to devolve down to local level

The results lead to six initiatives (see also *Improvement, expansion reform, 2003*):

1. every patient to have their own Health space on the internet
2. improvements in the range of primary care services
3. improvements in pharmacy services: increasing prescribing powers for non-medical staff; enhancing the power of pharmacists including helping patients manage minor ailments
4. reduce waiting lists and offer choice of providers
5. widen choice of treatment and care in maternity and terminal care: includes direct access to midwives and good care for the dying whatever the cause - not just for cancer and HIV/AIDS
6. improve quality and availability of information

Further reading:
Independent Midwives Association (2003) *A solution to the problem: IMA's submission to the Choice, Responsiveness and Equity Group.* London: IMA (see Midwifery chapter)

Department of Health (2003) *Improvement, expansion and reform: the next three years: priorities and planning framework.* London: Department of Health

Summary: directed at service managers, plans for health and social care include:

- offering patients more choice
- payment by results
- improving health and social care services for older people outside hospital
- rewarding organisations that perform well e.g. by offering foundation status

Tasks for trusts and other health organisations include: emergency planning; provision of good information to enable patients to share decision-making; ensure safety for patients; take into account the European working time directives (see above); provide for the training and development of staff; be involved in the new technology and communications systems

Department of Health (2003) *The Department of Health's change programme.* London: Department of Health

Summary: the Department is changing in line with the Prime Minister's four principles of public sector reform:

1. setting national standards
2. devolution of authority as far locally as possible
3. creating a diverse range of service providers
4. introducing and strengthening service users' power to choose

The Department's new structure comprises three business groups whose plans focus on organisation, leadership, people and communications.

- Health and Social Care Delivery Group
- Health and Social Care Standards and Quality Group
- Strategy and Business Development Group

Groups to be managed by a smaller management board comprising eight directors.

Chief Nursing Officer (2003) *Developing key roles for nurses and midwives: a guide for managers.* London: Department of Health

Summary: proposes enhanced and extended roles for nurses and midwives based on the *NHS plan's* aim to improve the patient experience. Illustrated with case studies, offers guidance for managers on introducing new roles whilst noting legal and professional boundaries. The key roles are: ordering diagnostic tests; making and receiving referrals; admitting and discharging patients; managing a caseload; running clinics; prescribing; resuscitation; minor procedures; triage and taking a lead in determining local services.

Department of Health (2003) *A vision for pharmacy in the new NHS.* London: Department of Health

Summary: focuses on five areas of improvement in community pharmacy services where people have most contact:

1. improve access by making more medicines available over the counter; allowing repeat prescriptions without a visit to GP, allowing direct referrals via NHS Direct; providing one-stop pharmacy advice; improving out-of-hours access; electronic prescribing
2. help patients manage their medication better
3. make pharmacy services patient-led by extending range of services; integrating with other out-of-hours services; giving pharmacists limited prescribing powers; improving hospital service so that patients can continue to use their medicines in hospital
4. improve safety and professional regulation, improving staff recruitment and retention
5. introduce a pharmacy service for prisons and other developments

Further reading:
Lewis, R. and Jenkins, C. (2002) *Community pharmacy: what pharmacists think is needed.* London: King's Fund

Department of Health (2003) *The NHS knowledge and skills framework and related development review.* London: The Stationery Office

Summary: designed to be used in conjunction with *Agenda for change (2004)* the KSF is designed to:

- identify the knowledge and skills that workers should apply in their post
- help to direct an individual's development
- provide a framework for review and professional development
- provide the basis for progression and increments in the pay scale

The framework comprises six core dimensions common to all posts, plus sixteen that will apply to some jobs but not others. Core dimensions are communication; personal and people development; health, safety and security; service development; quality and equality; diversity and rights. Most jobs incorporate the core, plus between three and six of the specific dimensions. Each dimension is further defined by level descriptors indicating successively more advanced knowledge and skill.

Development Review is an individual's professional review based on a four-stage adult learning cycle:

1. joint review between individual and line manager
2. production of personal development plan
3. learning and development to be supported by line manager
4. evaluation of learning and the application of what has been learnt

At set points on the pay band, pay increases will depend on individuals demonstrating applied knowledge and skills to a set level. 'Foundation gateways' relate to knowledge and skills required at the outset of appointment, 'second gateways' apply to someone fully developed in a post.

Further reading:
Benton, D.C. (2003) Agenda for change: the knowledge and skills framework. *Nursing Standard* 18(6) 33-9

Watts, A. and Green, S. (2004) Valuing your skills. *Nursing Management* 11(2) 16-7

Agenda for Change Project Team (2004) *Agenda for change: what will it mean for you?* London: Department of Health

Summary: due to roll out from December 2004 until September 2005 after a series of pilot schemes run in 2003, *Agenda for change* represents a radical new pay system for all NHS staff except doctors, dentists and the most senior managers.

- the system aims to offer equal pay for work of equal value; it opens the possibilities for creating new, more varied and stimulating posts; it aims to take away the pay ceiling and to make pay more fairly based on actual work evaluation

- the Job Evaluation Scheme will measure the skills, knowledge and responsibilities of each post and place it on a scale of Bands from one to nine. New employees on band five will rise two increments within that band in their first year that will be called 'preceptorship'. Afterwards, increments will be earned only as long as skills and knowledge are developed

- except when working unsocial hours, there will be one set of working terms and conditions for all staff including: a standard working week of 37 ½ hours; overtime paid to all staff except those in the higher salary bands, at time-and-a-half except for the eight Bank Holidays; annual leave will be set at 27 days plus the Bank Holidays.

Further reading:
Department of Health (2003) *The new NHS pay system: an overview.* London: Department of Health

Harding, M. L. (2004) Agenda for delay. *Health Service Journal* 114(5898) 42-3

Commission of the European Communities (2004) *Proposal for a directive of the European Parliament and of the Council amending directive 2003/88/EC concerning certain aspects of the organisation of working time.* Brussels: Commission of the European Communities

Summary: arises from the experience of applying the 1993 directive, in particular with the 'opt out' agreements and the impossibility of holding organisations to even a 58-hour week

- OPT-OUTs: employees were allowed to sign an opt-out agreement and in some countries, especially the UK, the agreement was presented at the same time as the employment contract. This shouldn't be allowed to continue and furthermore an employee should be allowed to withdraw his consent to opt- out at any time

- the SIMAP and Jaeger Judgements ruling that on-call time on the premises should be classed as working time, has proved financially untenable in many countries, especially in the health and social care sectors; some member states would have had to employ tens of thousands more medical staff

A new directive would attempt to find a balance between organisations' financial interests and the rights and safety of workers. They propose:

- OPT-OUTs: conditions associated with gaining an employee's consent should be much more stringent: the agreement must not be given at the same time as the employment contract; it must be in writing and should be valid for a year at a time, with no worker working longer than 65 hours per week, no matter what the circumstances

- ON-CALL time: would introduce 'inactive on-call' time which would not be considered working time although member states would have the option of counting it as such; rest periods may be calculated within every 72 hours instead of 24

Further reading:
Department of Health (2004) *A compendium of solutions to implementing the Working Time Directive for doctors in training from August 2004.* London: Department of Health

Department of Health (2004) *The NHS improvement plan: putting people a the heart of public services.* London: Department of Health

Summary: outlines priorities for the next four years. Progress so far includes huge budgetary increase from about £680 per capita in 1997 to £1345 in 2004. Staff levels are increasing and extensive modernisation and building plans are going on. Death rates from cancer stroke and heart disease are falling as are waiting lists for outpatient appointments and elective surgery. Proposed improvements include

- reduce waiting times further; from 2005 patients may determine when they are seen and choose from more than four providers and by 2008 any provider, as long as the cost comes within the national tariff
- patients to have access to their personal Health Space on the internet, that will show their care records and note their preferences
- more support for people with chronic illness such as diabetes, asthma and mental illnesses; an Expert Patient Programme will enable people to take control of their care, supported by a clinical team
- in public health, the white paper *Choosing health (2004)* will amongst other things look at further reducing deaths from cancer, stroke, heart disease and suicide
- hospital care: the Health Commission will take responsibility for inspection of all non-NHS providers
- in primary care, new teams to include GP specialists and community matrons
- by 2005 we can expect to see: electronic appointment booking; e-prescribing, electronic patient records and the Health Space
- by 2008: the 'payment by results' system will be fully installed; there will be financial incentives to support people with long-term illness; NHS foundation trusts will be fully operational, working free of Whitehall control

Further reading:
Audit Commission (2004) *Choice in public services.* London: Audit Commission

Supplementary Reading

Alberti, G. (2004) *Transforming emergency care in England.* London: Department of Health

Audit Commission (2001) *A spoonful of sugar: medicines management in NHS hospitals.* London: Audit Commission

Audit Commission (1992) *Making time for patients: a handbook for ward sisters.* London: HMSO

Coker, Naaz (ed) (2001) *Racism in medicine: an agenda for change.* London: King's Fund

Comptroller and Auditor General (2002) *NHS Direct in England.* (HC505 Session 2001-2002) London: The Stationery Office

Department of Health (2001) *The effective management of occupational health and safety services in the NHS.* London: Department of Health

Department of Health (2001) *National taskforce on violence against social care staff: report and national action plan.* London: The Stationery Office

Department of Health (1992) *Nurses, Midwives and Health Visitors Act 1992: chapter 16.* London: HMSO

Department of Health (1993) *Report on the taskforce on the strategy for research in nursing, midwifery and health visiting.* (chair Adrian Webb) London: Department of Health

Dewar, S. (2003) *Government and the NHS; time for a new relationship?* London: King's Fund

Harrabin R. et al (2003) *Health in the news: risk, reporting and media influence.* London: King's Fund

Harrison, Anthony (2001) *Making the right connections: the design and management of health care delivery.* London: King's Fund

Kingsley, Sue and Pawar, Asha (2002) *Putting race equality to work in the NHS: a resource for action.* London: Department of Health

National Audit Office (2004) *Improving emergency care in England: report by the Comptroller and Auditor General: HC1075 session 2003-04.* London: The Stationery Office

NHS Executive (2000) *Workforce and development: embodying leadership in the NHS.* London: NHSE

NHS Management Executive (1993) *A vision for the future: the nursing, midwifery and health visiting contribution to health and health care.* London: Department of Health

Nurses, Midwives and Health Visitors Act 1997: chapter 24. London: The Stationery Office

Performance and Innovation Unit, Cabinet Office (2001) *Strengthening leadership in the public sector: a research study.* London: PIU

Race Relations (Amendment) Act 2000: chapter 34. London: The Stationery Office

Regulatory Impact Unit, Cabinet Office (2002) *Making a difference: reducing burdens in hospitals.* London: Department of Health

Toynbee, Polly and Walker, David (2000) *Did things get better? An audit of Labour's successes and failures.* Harmondsworth: Penguin Books

Wright, S. (ed) (1993) *The named nurse, midwife and health visitor.* London: Department of Health

2 Quality

Parker, Roy (1990) *Safeguarding standards: a report on the desirability and feasibility of establishing a UK independent body to regulate and promote good practice in social work and social care.* London: National Institute for Social Work

Summary: a steering committee was set up in 1987 to consider establishing an independent body to regulate social work and social care: GSSC General Social Services Council. The Joseph Rowntree Memorial Trust funded this feasibility study following a report in 1982 that had judged the implementation of such a council as 'premature'. Changes in social services during the 80's strengthened the case for an independent council whereas there was no increase in the arguments against it.

Access to Health Records Act 1990: chapter 23. London: HMSO

Summary: allows a person to apply to view their patient records whether they are a) the patient b) an authorised adult acting on their behalf, c) a parent/guardian d) appointed to manage their affairs or in the event of a death e) a personal representative or someone who has claim as a result of that death. the record holder must allow the individual to inspect or have copies of the records, giving explanation where needed (e.g. medical terminology). The Act give circumstances where access might be denied and where it would be possible to amend incorrect details.

Department of Health (1991) *The patient's charter.* London HMSO

Summary: this launched the Conservative government's Citizen's Charter initiative in the specific area of the NHS and its standards. The forward stresses the importance of maintaining the tenets on which the NHS was originally founded, i.e. a service that is freely available to all at the point of need. The basic message is 'the patient comes first'. It invites views and suggestions from patients and also imposes an obligation on health authorities to provide information about its services. The 3 main sections are:

- existing patients' rights, i.e. access to health records and emergency care
- 3 new rights: information on local services and standards; guaranteed maximum 2-year waiting lists; full investigation and response to complaints
- 9 national charter standards such as: respect for religious beliefs; minimum waiting times for ambulances; assessment in accident and emergency departments and the introduction of the "named nurse" concept.

Further reading:
Cohen, P. (1994) Passing the buck?...Patient's charter seems to have raised the expectations of people using the health service. *Nursing Times* 90(13) 28-30

Shuttleworth, A. (1992) Will the charter work? Readers views on the Patient's charter. *Professional Nurse* 7(7) 439-41

Department of Health (1995) *The patient's charter and you.* London: Department of Health

Summary: expanded and updated version of the *Patient's charter (1991).* Sets out patients' rights and standards of service they can expect to receive. Distinguishes between rights which all patients will receive all the time; and expectations which are standards of service which the NHS is aiming to achieve. Areas looked at are:

- rights and standards throughout the NHS e.g. access to services
- GP services e.g. registering with and changing doctors
- hospital services e.g. reducing waiting times
- community services e.g. appointment times
- ambulance services e.g. ambulance arrival times
- dental, optical and pharmaceutical services
- outlines how patients can help the NHS by using its services responsibly e.g. by returning equipment

Further reading:
Friend, B. (1995) Shallow standards: pressure to meet Patient's Charter targets means that some hospitals are fiddling the figures. *Nursing Times* 91(28) 14-5

Ryland, R.K. (1996) The Patients' Charter: the United Kingdom experience. *Journal of Advanced Nursing* 23(6) 1059-60

Farrell, Christine (1998) *The patient's charter: past and future.* London: King's Fund

Harding, Tessa and Beresford, Peter (1996) *The standards we expect: what service users and carers want from social services workers.* London: National Institute for Social Work

Summary: this report forms part of a study on standards commissioned by the Department of Health. The people involved represented a wide cross-section of voluntary and user-controlled organisations across the country and welcomed the opportunity to contribute to setting standards of practice. The main points that arose were:

- making involvement possible, including a more 'child-friendly' forum that would enable children to voice their needs in a less daunting setting
- making standards stick - across the board standards were viewed as inconsistent. Standards should not merely exist on paper but be enforceable in practice. Monitoring and improving standards should be ongoing with people called to account if they do not meet the standards
- making standards consistent - common standards should be applied across health and social services and also across children's services and education

The final report falls into 4 parts covering the quality of relationships; the quality of skills; the quality of services and areas for improvement with plans for action.

Caldicott Committee: Department of Health (1997) *Report on the review of patient identifiable information.* (chair Fiona Caldicott) London: Department of Health

Summary: the review was commissioned because of the development of information technology that has allowed patient information to be disseminated widely and quickly. The 16 recommendations include:

- to strengthen the awareness of the need for confidentiality and security
- organisations to appoint 'guardians' responsible for safeguarding confidentiality
- there must be protocols written about the exchange of information and access to patient identity
- a NHS number to replace all other identifiers as soon as possible
- health and information systems to incorporate best principles at the design stage
- GP claims and payments to avoid transmission of patients' details

Further reading:
Barber, Barry (1998) How should we treat personal medical data. *British Journal of Healthcare Computing and Information Management* 15(1) 23-26

Walker, Phil (1998) Caldicott implementation: protecting and using confidential patient information in the modern NHS. *British Journal of Healthcare Computing and Information Management* 15(7) 28-30

Wells, Mike (1998) Caldicott guardians and the NHS strategic tracing service. *British Journal of Healthcare Computing and Information Management* 15(7) 32-35

Department of Health (1998) *A first class service: quality in the new NHS.* London: Department of Health

Summary: consultation document focusing on improving quality standards, efficiency, openness and accountability. The Government proposes:

- a National Institute for Clinical Excellence (NICE) which will assess new and existing interventions for their clinical and cost-effectiveness and produce national guidance for clinicians and patients
- National Service Frameworks will lay down the care that different groups of patients may expect to receive in major care areas or disease groups such as older people and cancer

These standards will be applied locally through a system of clinical governance, extended life-long learning and professional self-regulation. Standards will be monitored through three new mechanisms:

- a Commission for Health Improvement
- a National Framework for Assessing Performance
- an annual National Survey of Patient and User Experience

Further reading:
Coulter, A. (1999) *NICE and CHI: reducing variations and raising standards.* London: King's Fund

Crinson, Iain (1999) Clinical governance: the new NHS, new responsibilities. *British Journal of Nursing* 8(7) 449-53

Walshe, K. (1998) Going first class with the NHS. *Health Service Journal* 108(5612) 18-19

NHS Executive (1998) *In the public interest: developing a strategy for public participation in the NHS.* London: The Stationery Office

Summary: this report looks at the public's involvement in decision-making for health provision in the new NHS and in the light of greater access to information generally. The rationale and ethical considerations for public participation are discussed in the first two sections. Four models of participation are outlined in the third and fourth sections:

- direct participation of users
- informed view of citizens
- community development
- local scrutiny and accountability

The final section gives recommendations for health policy in relation to NHS staff such as improved dissemination of information, the role of primary care groups and partnerships with other agencies.

Further reading:
Ainsworth, Steve (1998) Voices of dissent. *Health Service Journal* 108(5618) 23

NHS Executive (1998) *Information for health: an information strategy for the modern NHS 1998-2005.* London: NHSE

Summary: the aim is to ensure that information is used "to help patients receive the best possible care. The means improving access for both patients and health professionals." Key objectives are:

- electronic patient records with 24-hour access for primary and acute sector
- a computerised infrastructure that will enable delivery of electronic information via NHS Net
- ensuring good quality information is brought together and made accessible to support clinical governance. This includes setting up the National Electronic Library for Health
- develop the informatics skills of health professionals and managers
- establish NHS Direct as a telephone and internet helpline

Implementation requires close cooperation at national and local level and considerable financial support. Finance will come from the Spending Review Modernisation Fund: more than £1 billion between 1998 and 2005.

Further reading:
National Audit Office (2002) *NHS Direct in England: report by the Comptroller and Auditor General: HC505 session 2001-02.* London: The Stationery Office

Department of the Environment, Transport and the Regions, and Department of Health (1999) *Better care, higher standards: a charter for long term care.* London: The Stationery Office

Summary: designed to encourage the cooperation of local health, housing and social services, in order to help users of long term care, and to improve services to them. The charter is aimed at anyone over 18 with long term care needs, and their carers. It sets standards for the services provided by local health, housing and social service departments. These standards are published in local charters that should be widely available from June 2000; information is also given about what to do when services fall below the standard. The six main areas are:

- providing information to users and carers about the services available
- understanding and responding to the needs of users and carers
- finding suitable living accommodation
- promoting and helping with independent living
- receiving appropriate health care
- assisting carers

The charter will help to ensure consistency across the country: elements of the charter are already in place in some areas, but not all. Finally, users and carers are reminded that they also have a part to play in achieving good outcomes, the charter encourages them to:

- give full information
- keep appointments
- keep service providers up-to-date with their needs
- follow medical advice about treatment and medication
- look after equipment
- tell service providers what they might do to improve their services

Department of Health (1999) *Supporting doctors, protecting patients: a consultation paper on preventing, recognising and dealing with poor clinical performance of doctors in the NHS in England.* London: Department of Health

Summary: a paper that arises from *A first class service (1998)* and the recent inquiries into medical malpractice. The common themes to arise from recent cases have been: a pattern of poor practice over a long period; problems known about but not officially; the failure of systems that were set up to detect problems. Proposals include:

- improving professional self-regulation and accountability
- the clinical governance programme to ensure a thorough review of quality
- measures involving education, supervision and stress relief to prevent problems occurring in the first place

For handling and dealing with problems, 3 steps are identified:

1. identifying which category it falls into i.e.: personal misconduct, serious mistake or others' concerns about clinical performance

2. setting up Assessment and Support Centres around the country

3. employer or health authority to take responsibility for carrying out the findings of the Assessment and Support Centres; Health Authorities to have the power to suspend general practitioners.

Further reading:

Chief Medical Officer (2001) *Harold Shipman's clinical practice, 1974 - 1998.* (chair Richard Baker) London: The Stationery Office

Hill, A.P. and Baeza, Juan (1999) Dealing with things that go wrong. *Lancet* 354(9196) 2099-10

Hutchinson, Martin (2000) Will regulation reforms help doctors improve? *Hospital Doctor* 20.1.00 30-33

Jewell, D. (2000) Supporting doctors, or the beginning of the end for self-regulation? *British Journal of General Practice* 50(450) 4-5

Department of Health (1999) *Code of practice on openness in the NHS.* London: NHS Executive

Summary: addressed to trusts and health authorities the code is based on the principle that the NHS is a public service and as such it's workings should be transparent, with information about how it works openly available to the public. Points include:

*   access to information about services, costs, quality and performance
*   notice of proposed changes, with opportunities to respond and influence decisions
*   patient access to health records as well as the reasoning behind their treatments
*   NHS to be prompt in response to requests for information, making sure there are clear arrangements for dealing with complaints
*   outlines rare instances where information may be withheld or charged for
*   the specific obligations of PCTs, health authorities, dentists, community pharmacists, optometrists and GPs

Brand, Don (1999) *Accountable care: developing the General Social Care Council.* London: Joseph Rowntree Foundation

Summary: this describes how the notion of standard setting in social care evolved since 1990 with a General Social Care Council (GSCC) proposed in 1993. Comparing councils in England, Scotland and Wales, the main principles that emerge are to do with empowering and protecting users, with a strong user representation and 'open' working. A survey of user organisations reveals a confidence in the GSCC provided it is fully responsive to users and not remote or bureaucratic. Staff contracts will include codes of conduct and staff are content with this, provided there is strong support and access to training. On the other hand, employers must have defined expectations in recruitment, supervision and management and there must be a code of practice for handling complaints and disciplinaries.

Further reading:
Department of Health (1996) *Obligations of care: a consultation paper on the setting of conduct and practice standards for social services staff.* London: Department of Health

Harding, Tessa and Beresford, Peter (1996) *Standards we expect: what service users and carers want from social services departments.* London: National Institute for Social Work

Parker, R. A. (1990) *Safeguarding standards.* London: National Institute for Social Work

Department of Health (2000) *A quality strategy for social care.* London: The Stationery Office

Summary: the strategy builds on *Modernising social services (1998)*; it outlines the reforms required in working practices and the training and management needed to improve the quality of social services. Across the country social services should:

- promote independence
- strengthen families by supporting parental responsibility
- improve the life chances of children in need
- tackle inequality and social exclusion

There are too many failings in the system however, due to bureaucracy, inflexibility, poor coordination, inadequately trained staff, and inconsistent service delivery from one area to another. The aims of the strategy therefore are to:

- tackle inconsistency
- create a new Social Care Institute for Excellence to convert evidence-based knowledge into quality practice
- introduce a new Quality Framework to help local councils improve the quality of their social care service
- improve workforce training at all levels from management down

Further reading:
Editorial (2001) Raising the standard of social care in England. *Professional Social Work* January 2001 6-7

Statham, D. (2000) Look and learn. *Community Care* 5.10.01 24

Department of Health (2000) *Improving working lives standard: NHS employers committed to improving the working lives of people who work in the NHS.* London: Department of Health

Summary: the result of a consultation exercise with NHS staff, trade unions and the Royal Colleges. Employers are expected to offer flexible working that will protect and support staff. Other statements include:

- the need for a modern employment service
- staff's right to a balance between work and home life
- working arrangements that find a balance between patient needs and what staff are able to provide
- staff to feel valued for their commitment
- staff's right to personal and professional development

£25,000 has been offered to every trust for staff to spend as they wish on improving the working environment. Between £6 and £8 million to be invested over three years in extending occupational health services to general practice staff. £140 million has gone towards training and development for all staff and £30 million invested in childcare support. The standard should be in place by April 2003 with implementation in three stages that will be kite-marked:

1. Pledge - organisation putting the framework in place
2. Practice - putting policies into practice
3. Practice plus - achievement in all staff groups by 2006

Further reading:
Millar, B. (2001) Behind every great nurse. *Nursing Times* 97(12) 24-6

Department of Health (2000) *An organisation with a memory: report of an expert group on learning from adverse events in the NHS.* (chair Chief Medical Officer) London: The Stationery Office

Summary: the report claims the NHS often fails to learn from adverse events and has an old fashioned approach when compared with other sectors. A fundamental review would provide many benefits in terms of saving lives, preventing harm and freeing up much needed resources. To this end the report recommends:

*   a unified mechanism for report and analysis when things go wrong
*   a more open working culture so as to encourage the reporting of errors and discourages individual scapegoating
*   a mechanism for making sure that recommended changes are put into practice
*   a wider appreciation of the 'value system' approach to learning from errors

Further reading:
Scott, Helen (2000) Individuals must not take the blame for the system. *British Journal of Nursing* 9(12) 744

Sommerville, Fiona (2000) Systems fail, not just individuals. *Nursing Standard* 96(32) 23

Department of Health (2000) *Your guide to the NHS.* London: Department of Health

Summary: published after the *NHS plan (2000)*, in all but name this is a third edition of *The patients' charter 1991*. It sets out what patients may expect from the NHS as well as what is promised over the next five years.

*   begins by stating the ten core principles of the NHS including that it should be free to all at the point of need and that it aims to be needs-led, seamless and working to a consistently high standard
*   lists patients' responsibilities to themselves - including tips for healthy living - and to the service
*   explains the functions of the different agencies such as NHS Direct, general practitioners, pharmacists etc

Planned improvements include:
- further development of NHS Direct
- promises to do with waiting times and cancellations
- improvements in standards of hygiene and quality of meals
- greater patient representation and involvement in the planning of services

Department of Health (2001) *Establishing the new Nursing and Midwifery Council.* London: Department of Health

Summary: this sets out the plan to replace the UKCC and the 4 national boards with a Nursing and Midwifery Council and a single professional register. Main aims:
- patient welfare paramount
- faster, more 'transparent' working procedures
- accountability to the health service and to the public
- the Council to have wider powers to regulate dangerous individuals
- Council to be smaller, elected and with a strong lay representation
- explicit powers to link registration with evidence of professional development

Main changes include:
- a president, first appointed through open competition and then elected by Council
- each member to have a 'seconder' to attend meetings and vote in their absence
- a statutory midwifery committee
- wider powers to pay fees and allowances in order to secure the highest possible calibre of membership
- NMC to be accountable to Privy Council instead of the Secretary of State
- Government to have the power set up inquiries into the NMC's performance

Further reading:
Drazek, M (2000) The new Nursing and Midwifery Council: what does modernising mean for midwives. *Practising Midwife* 3(9) 10-2

Duffin, C. (2001) Taking change on board...the metamorphosis of the UKCC to the Nursing and Midwifery Council. *Nursing Standard* 15(23) 12-3

Department of Health (2001) *Building a safer NHS for patients.* London: Department of Health

Summary: a plan to promote patient safety, the key points are:
- standardising the definition and system for reporting adverse events - this leading to an international standard
- a National Patient Safety Agency to collect, analyse and feed back data on adverse events; providing information about safety and producing solutions and national goals

- the system for handling investigations to be either through a Department of Health commission or the Commission for Health Improvement only. Major service failures may lead to a public inquiry led by the Secretary of State for Health
- specific targets include: to reduce to nil the number of patients dying or paralysed by poorly administered spinal injections, to reduce instances of harm in obstetrics and gynaecology and to reduce errors in the use of prescription drug
- to develop the evidence base on patient safety

Department of Health (2001) *Information for social care: a framework for improving quality in social care through better use of information and information technology.* London: The Stationery Office

Summary: information plays a crucial part in the delivery of high quality social care services; sometimes information is the service itself since users need information on what is available and Central Government needs information in order to keep track of performance. This document provides a toolkit for councils, the Department of Health and other partner agencies can use to tackle information management. It presents a detailed overview of the main issues i.e.:

- the electronic social care record
- knowledge management
- access and communication channels
- infrastructure
- culture
- funding
- planning and project management

Audit Commission (2003) *Human rights: improving public service delivery.* London: Audit Commission

Summary: a report that considers the implications of the *Human Rights Act 1998* for public services, citing examples of progress and good practice and demonstrating how the Act can be used as a framework for development. It stresses the importance of responding to the Act because:

- it is the law to protect the rights of individuals
- it can improve services, in particular for users with mental health and learning disability issues
- the cost of not responding to the Act is high, not only financially but also to the reputation of the organisation

Department of Health (2003) *NHS complaints reform: making things right.* London: Department of Health

Summary: the result of a listening exercise and two-year evaluative study this plan hopes to:

- change the way people view complaints so that the professional - patient relationship improves and so that complaints may be seen as an opportunity to examine and improve that area of service
- make handling complaints a normal part of managing a service
- make CHAI and CSCI responsible for handling the independent review stage
- use what is learnt from mistakes as a normal part of the audit process and a system that is constantly improving

The Commission for Healthcare Audit and Inspection and the Commission for Social Care Inspection to become fully operational in April 2004. Both must establish a complaints function in alignment with each other. The plan also provides for training, new legislation, the development of the Patient Advisory Liaison Service (PALS) and for the Modernisation Agency to develop PCTs' and Strategic Health Authorities' complaints handling.

Health and Social Care (Community Health and Standards) Act 2003: chapter 43. London: The Stationery Office

Summary: provides for the creation of NHS Foundation trusts and for independent healthcare and social care regulators namely the Commission for Healthcare Audit and Inspection (CHAI) and the Commission for Social Care Inspection (CSCI). Also:

- provides for the NHS to recover treatment costs where people receive compensation for injuries
- places a duty on primary care trusts to provide or 'secure delivery' of primary dental and medical services, making 'permanent' previously piloted personal medical services agreements
- replaces of the Welfare Food scheme that had originally been set up for mothers and newborns at a time of rationing

Department of Health and Chief Medical Officer (2003) *Making amends: a consultation setting out proposals for reforming the approach to clinical negligence in the NHS.* London: Department of Health

Summary: describes how matters can go wrong, leading to serious consequences for a patient. The commonest reasons for complaint are: death, pain, missed diagnosis and medication error. In hospitals most claims are in the surgical and obstetric/ gynaecology specialties. A full explanation is needed with an apology and where appropriate, financial compensation. Current medical litigation costs are enormous with not enough getting to the patient. The system is complex, slow and unfair leaving the patient dissatisfied and doctors demoralised, encouraging them to practice defensive medicine. There should instead be an emphasis on reducing risk and bringing down the number of errors that occur by learning from mistakes. The UK NHS is almost the first in the world to look systematically at risk and patient safety. This paper makes the following recommendations:

- establish a NHS Redress Scheme to investigate and explain error and offer a package of care, not just financial compensation
- NHS Litigation Authority to oversee the work of the Redress Scheme and arrange finance
- standards of care should include complaints management
- each trust to appoint an individual at board level to take responsibilities for adverse events
- effective rehabilitation should be offered where appropriate
- all neurologically impaired and physically disabled children should have access to special care within the NHS
- there should be a duty of candour on the part of clinicians
- consider mediation before litigation

Further reading:

Allen, T. (2003) Making amends: mediating medical matters. *British Journal of Health Care Management* 9(9) 301-4

Tingle, J. (2003) Making amends: reforming the clinical negligence system. *Health Care Risk Report* 9(8) 10-11

National Audit Office (2003) *The management of suspensions of clinical staff in NHS hospital and ambulance trusts in England: report by the Comptroller and Auditor General: HC1143 session 2002-3.* London: The Stationery Office

Summary: 1000 members of staff were suspended/excluded in year 2001-2 for an average 47 weeks for doctors and nineteen weeks for others. About 200 of those were doctors of whom more than 40% returned to work. Reasons for exclusion were incompetence or professional or personal misconduct. The total cost was £29m, the cost of excluding clinicians - £11m. The average cost of excluding a doctor is £188,00, of others - £21,000. The report suggests that if exclusions could be completed within 24 weeks the NHS would make a saving of £14m. Detailed recommendations for the Department of Health and the Trusts look at speeding up the process, reviewing causes to protect patients and avoid repeating mistakes.

Department of Health and Information Policy Unit (2003) *Confidentiality: NHS code of practice.* London: Department of Health

Summary: aimed at all NHS staff but in particular, Caldicott Guardians and data protection officers, the code runs as follows:

1. defines confidentiality
2. describes how a service should appear
3. explains the law and how it should apply within the health service

4. proposes a decision-making tool for managing disclosure of information

5. offers scenario-based examples of good practice

Strategic Health Authorities and the Commission for Healthcare Audit and Inspection to play a key role in ensuring all parts of the NHS are running effective systems.

National Audit Office (2003) *Achieving improvements through clinical governance: a progress report on implementation by NHS Trusts: report by the Comptroller and Auditor General: HC1055 session 2002-3.* London: The Stationery Office

Summary: reiterates the principles of clinical governance as:

- a coherent approach to quality improvement
- setting clear lines of accountability
- establishing processes for identifying and managing risk and poor performance

Since 1997 the NHS is on a ten-year programme setting clear national standards via the National Service Frameworks and NICE guidelines with local delivery ensured by the NHS Modernisation Agency and effective monitoring carried out by the Strategic Health Authorities (SHA) and the Commission for Health Improvement (CHI). the report focuses on secondary and tertiary care and findings include:

- structures are in place
- quality has become a mainstream issue with open accountability, transparent working and some improvements in practice and patient care
- progress in implementing clinical governance is patchy between trusts and between components within trusts
- trusts need more support; 43% of trusts have had valued help from Clinical Governance Support Teams (CGST)
- most funding comes from within trusts with little back-up from SHAs or PCTs
- external review such as from CHI have made things happen although progress feels slow and SHAs should work to ensure action is 'timely'
- progress has happened where there is a statutory or external requirement but not merely desirable such as with knowledge management or patient and public involvement

Recommendations to the Department of Health and Trusts include:

- CGSTs to disseminate examples of good practice
- DoH to draw up guidelines for patient empowerment and consider rewarding trusts for progress
- CHI (soon to be CHAI) inspections should include questions about workers' attitudes to and experience of clinical governance, identifying barriers and proposing solutions
- trusts to ensure provision of good information, reporting on quality issues and drawing up annual plans and programmes for development
- ensure open, transparent working and share good practice

Further reading:
Donaldson, L. and Halligan, A. (2001) Implementing clinical governance: turning vision into reality. *British Medical Journal* 322 1413-17

Department of Health (2003) *Raising standards: improving performance in the NHS.* London: Department of Health

Summary: the Government wants all NHS hospitals working to a consistently high standard so that by 2008, they may apply for foundation status. The Government also wants PCTs to be strong and capable of commissioning services according to the needs of their communities. Responsibility for this rests with Trusts supported by Government, Strategic Health Authorities and the NHS Modernisation Agency. Proposes a four-point programme aimed at two-star trusts or lower:

- clear assessment
- tailored support from the Modernisation Agency
- develop leadership
- targeted resources: £200m available between years 04/5 and 07/8 to implement local improvement

The Government's role to support this involves:

- sustained investment with three-year allocations so that trusts can plan with confidence
- building and modernisation programme
- developments in information technology to support electronic booking, integrated electronic patient records, digital imaging and electronic prescribing
- publishing clear standards via NSFs and NICE guidelines
- modernising the workforce
- working towards devolved authority
- promoting patient empowerment through providing good information and choice about when and where they can be treated
- NHS Modernisation Agency working since 2001 to spread good practice and promote leadership
- measuring performance via the Commission for Healthcare Audit and Inspection and the Commission for Social Care Inspection

So far improvements can be seen in:

- reduced waiting times for outpatient appointments and surgery
- increased staff levels
- deaths from cancer and heart disease are falling

Commission for Health Improvement (2003) *Getting better? a report on the NHS.* London: The Stationery Office

Summary: based on CHI's findings from 250 reviews of hospitals and other NHS organisations in England and Wales. Notes that CHI has only been going for three years and that these reviews have not covered all of the NHS yet (e.g. few PCTs) Nevertheless feels markers of a successful service include:

- effective treatment
- quick easy-to-use service
- well-organised service
- being treated with dignity and respect
- surroundings that are clean, safe and comfortable

Factors that are crucial to improvement include: good leadership that drives progress; clear policies and plans; integrated staff working; a reflective organisation that learns from experience - good and bad; education and training and cooperation with other agencies. Where they see improvements in the NHS compared with ten years ago:

- NSFs and guidelines are leading to more consistent services
- waiting times are getting shorter
- staff levels are increasing slowly
- there is progress in involving patients in decision-making
- building projects and improvements to existing premises
- greater opportunities for staff development
- more paramedics and even volunteers have been trained to use defibrillators
- where large numbers of psychiatric patients would be 'put away' in the past, some mental health trusts now lead the field in advocacy and in involving patients and carers in planning their treatment and care in the community. Improvements are not yet on a large enough scale to affect the majority of users. Services are 'patchy and inconsistent' with pockets of good care not mirrored by the rest of the organisation. Some areas are getting worse with poor services and environments in mental health compared with hospital services.

Department of Health (2004) *Standards for better health.* London: The Stationery Office

Summary: aimed at NHS and Social Services, this comes as part of a three-year plan *National standards, local action (2004)* and stresses the need to focus on health outcomes and patient experience. Sets out standards to ensure services are safe and of good quality as well as providing for continuous improvement and best use of the newly invested money. This is also an attempt to rationalise and simplify standard-setting mechanisms and reporting requirements from the past. The standards have 2 facets: 'core' and 'developmental' and are directed at all services in every care setting at every level. They are arranged to a structure of seven domains:

1. safety
2. clinical and cost effectiveness
3. governance
4. patient focus
5. accessible, responsive care
6. environment and amenities
7. public health

National Service Frameworks will continue to be developed and should be seen as part of 'developmental' standards. The work of the inspection agencies' - the Commission for Healthcare Audit and Inspection CHAI and the Commission for Social Care Inspection CSCI - is outlined; their reviews will contribute to future target making and planning.

Meredith, V. for Department of Health (2004) *Getting over the wall: how the NHS is improving the patient's experience.* London: Department of Health

Summary: a report with examples from around the country about making the NHS a patient/needs-led service and making patient and involvement a driving force in improvement. Whilst trusts are listening to patients and inviting their comments, those findings aren't then worked into decision-making. Where the process works, communities have a say in how resources are spent and patients a say in their own care. The report stresses the importance of the knowledge that patients bring to the process as well as the value of sharing information between decision-makers and the public. Too often however, patients feel they are being 'done to' and that there's a 'hidden agenda' that they are not party to. The report highlights how changes can be made by building on small successes e.g. taking care to control one's use of language.

Further reading:
Commission for Health Improvement (2004) *Unpacking the patients' perspective: variations in NHS patient experience in England.* London: CHI

NHS and National Patient Safety Agency (2004) *Seven steps to patient safety.* London: NPSA

Summary: aimed at all staff in England and Wales, particularly those responsible for risk management and clinical governance. Arises from recommendations made in *An organisation with a memory (2000),* the seven steps are:

1. promote a safety culture
2. lead and support staff
3. risk and management
4. encourage the reporting of incidents
5. nurture good communications with patients and the public
6. learn from mistakes and share the lessons learnt into order to:
7. put changes and improvements from lessons learnt into practice

Further reading:
National Patient Safety Agency (2003) Patient safety: seven steps to safety: the practice and policy that should be on your agenda. *Health Service Journal Supplement 113(5881) 1-13*

Supplementary reading:

Audit Commission (2002) *Data remember: improving the quality of patient-based information in the NHS.* London: Audit Commission

Commission for Health Improvement (2001) *A guide to clinical governance reviews in NHS acute trusts.* London: Commission for Health Improvement

Data Protection Registrar (1998) *Data Protection Act 1998: an introduction.* Cheshire: Wilmslow

Department of Health (1994) *Being heard: the report of a review committee on NHS complaints procedures.* London: Department of Health

Department of Health (2001) *The essence of care: patient-focused benchmarking for health care practitioners.* London: Department of Health

Department of Health (2001) *Extending choice for patients: a discussion document: proposals for pilot schemes to improve choice and provide faster treatment.* London: Department of Health

Department of Health (2000) *An inquiry into the quality and practice within the NHS arising from the actions of Rodney Ledward.* (chair Jean Ritchie) London: Department of Health

Department of Health (1999) *Patient and public involvement in the new NHS.* London: Department of Health

Dyke, Greg (1998) *The new NHS charter: a different approach: report on the new NHS charter.* London: Department of Health

Francis, S. et al (2003) *Improving the patient experience: evaluation of the King's Fund 'Enhancing the healing environment' programme.* London: The Stationery Office

General Medical Council 'Maintaining good medical practice' [WWW] http://www.gmc-uk.org/standards/MGMP.htm (17.11.04)

Harrison, A. (2003) *Getting the right medicines: putting public interest at the heart of health related research.* London: King's Fund

Herxheimer, A. et al (2000) Database of patient experiences: DIPex: a multimedia approach to sharing experiences and information. *Lancet* 355(9214) 1540-3

House of Commons (2003) *Needle Stick Injury Bill.* London: The Stationery Office

National Audit Office (2003) *A safer place to work: improving the management of health and safety risks to staff in NHS trusts: report by the Comptroller and Auditor General: HC623: session 2002-3.* London: The Stationery Office

National Audit Office (2003) *A safer place to work: protecting NHS hospital and ambulance staff from violence and aggression: report by the Comptroller and Auditor General: HC527: session: 2002-3.* London: The Stationery Office

National Audit Office (2003) *Safety, quality, efficacy: regulating medicines in the UK: report by the Comptroller and Auditor General: HC255 session 2002-3.* London: The Stationery Office

National Consumer Council (1999) *Involving users in the delivery of local public services.* London: NCC

National Consumer Council (1999) *Self-regulation of professionals in health care: consumer issues.* London: NCC

NHS (2001) *A commitment to quality, a quest for excellence: a statement on behalf of the Government, the medical profession and the NHS.* London: Department of Health

NHS Executive (1996) *Promoting clinical effectiveness: a framework for action in and through the NHS.* London: NHSE

NHS Executive (1999) *Clinical governance: quality in the new NHS.* London: NHSE

Nursing and Midwifery Council (2004) *Code of professional conduct: standards for conduct, performance and ethics.* London: NMC

Nursing and Midwifery Council (2004) *Guidelines for records and record-keeping.* London: NMC

Nursing and Midwifery Council (2004) *Guidelines for the administration of medicines.* London: NMC

Public Sector Inspection Team, Cabinet Office (2002) *Making a difference: reducing burdens in healthcare inspection and monitoring.* London: Department of Health

Royal College of General Practitioners (1999) *Clinical governance: practical advice for primary care in England and Wales.* London: RCGP

Royal College of Nursing (2000) *Clinical Governance: guidance for nurses.* London: RCN

3 Public Health

Department of Health (1992) *The health of the nation: a strategy for health in England (cm1986).* London: HMSO

Summary: the aim is to secure improvements in the general health of the population of England with the emphasis on disease prevention and health promotion. Aims to add years to life by increasing life expectancy and reducing premature death; and add life to years by increasing years lived free from ill health; reducing and minimising adverse effects of illness and disability; promoting healthy lifestyles and healthy physical and social environments; and improving the quality of life overall. Five key areas selected for action:

- Cancers
- Coronary heart disease and stroke
- Mental illness
- HIV/AIDS and sexual health
- Accidents

Each key area has overall objectives for improved health and specific targets to be met with emphasis placed on risk factors e.g. smoking. Recognises that targets cannot be met by NHS alone and advocates development of 'healthy alliances' between organisations such as local authorities and health authorities and individuals to work together to improve health. Sets out how the strategy will be monitored, reviewed and developed.

Further reading:

George, M. (1992) The health of the nation. *Nursing Standard* 6(44) 18-9

Harris, A. and Shapiro, J. (1994) Purchasers, professionals and public health: a need for a more radical appraisal of roles. *British Medical Journal* 308(6926) 426-7

Lawrence, M. (1992) Caring for the future. *British Medical Journal* 305(6850) 400-2

Whitty, Paula and Jones, Ian (1992) Public health heresy: a challenge to the purchasing orthodoxy. *British Medical Journal* 6833(304) 1039-41

Department of Health (1998) *Our healthier nation: a contract for health (cm3852).* London: The Stationery Office

Summary: consultative document on public health with two key aims:

1. 'Improve the health of the population as a whole by increasing the length of people's lives and the number of years people spend free from illness'.

2. 'Improve the health of the worst off in society and to narrow the health gap'.

   To achieve these two aims the Government proposes a 'national contract for better health' in which government, local communities and individuals will work together to improve health. The Government proposals include working internationally to improve health, ensuring that all national policies take full account of health, informing the public of health risks and the information they require to improve their health. Health authorities will have a key role in the development of local Health Improvement Programmes and will be expected to work closely with local authorities, primary care groups and local organisations. Health Action Zones will be set up and a network of Healthy Living Centres will be developed. The Government identifies four key targets to be achieved by 2010:

- heart disease and stroke - reduce the death rate by one-third in people under 65
- accidents - reduce by one-fifth
- cancer - reduce the death rate by one-fifth amongst people under 65
- mental health - reduce the death rate by one-sixth

Further reading:

Allen, D. (1998) Public health for all. *Community Practitioner* 71(3) 12-13

Moore, A. (1998) Target practice. *Nursing Standard* 12 (35) 24-25

Moores, Y. (1998) Nursing the patient better. *Nursing Times* 94(14) 36-37

Peckham, S. (1998) The missing link. *Health Service Journal* 108(5606) 22-23

Pickersgill, F. (1998) Nursing solutions. *Nursing Standard* 12 (42) 26-27

Department of Health (1998) *Independent inquiry into inequalities in health.* (chair Donald Acheson) London: The Stationery Office

Summary: this inquiry was carried out to influence health policy. The report identifies socioeconomic factors and lifestyle as crucial to health well-being. Some of the key areas include poverty, unemployment, housing, nutrition, families, ethnic and gender inequalities and disability. There are 39 recommendations listed at the end, many of which have implications for government policy. It is suggested that policies on education, employment, social services and other areas are constantly assessed and improved with health in mind. The last three of these relate to some of the areas covered in *NHS: modern, dependable (1998)* and *Our healthier nation (1998)* about equity of access and services and cooperation between health and social services.

Further reading:

Allen, D. (1999) Back in the Black. *Community Practitioner* 72(2) 11-12

Head, J. (2002) *Work environment, alcohol consumption and ill health: the Whitehall II study.* London: Health and Safety Executive

Townsend, Peter and Davidson, Nick (1982) *Inequalities in health: the Black report.* (chair Douglas Black) Harmondsworth: Penguin

Department of Health (1999) *Saving lives: our healthier nation (cm4386).* London: The Stationery Office

Summary: a white paper that grew out of *Our healthier nation (1998)* and *Independent inquiry into inequalities in health (1998).* An action plan with responsibilities for the public, community care services and the Government that sets targets to reduce death rates in cancer, heart disease, stroke, accidents and mental health to be achieved by the year 2010, saving 300,000 lives. As well as a commitment to the proposals made in *Our healthier nation (1998),* initiatives include:

- 'health skills' and 'expert patient' programmes to help people manage their health and illnesses
- tackling poverty and unemployment
- tackling smoking, sexual health, food safety, drugs and alcohol use, fluoridation and communicable diseases
- improving public health through a health development agency and a public health development fund

Further reading:

Baker, M.R. (2000) *Making sense of the new NHS white papers. 2e* Oxford: Radcliffe Medical Press

Crail, Mark (1999) Watching expiry dates. *Health Service Journal* 109(5663) 9-11

National Audit Office (2001) *Tackling obesity in England: report by the Comptroller and Auditor General.* London: The Stationery Office

Summary: since 1980, obesity has trebled in England and has serious implications in terms of contributing to disease, premature mortality and considerable financial consequences for the NHS. Findings:

- over half the women of this country and two thirds of men are either overweight or obese
- obesity can lead to: heart disease, type-2 diabetes, high blood pressure and osteoarthritis
- estimated cost to the NHS: £1/2 billion a year
- the main reasons for the increase are a combination of less active lifestyles, and changes in eating patterns, i.e. an excess of energy intake over expenditure

Because this is a lifestyle issue, there are limited ways for policy to affect changes, however recommendations include:

- cross-government initiatives in the areas of education, physical activity and diet, largely targeted at school children
- NICE and the Department of Health need to develop guidelines for the management of overweight and obese patients in primary care - the report gives an initial guide for general practitioners
- Health Authorities to develop Health Improvement Programmes that involve partner agencies in schemes to increase physical activity and improve diet
- an appendix lists 19 policies and initiatives that address the problem of obesity

Further reading:

Wardle, J. and Griffith, J. (2001) Socioeconomic status and weight control practices in British adults. *Journal of Epidemiology and Community Health* 55(3) 185-190

World Health Organisation (2000) *Obesity: preventing and managing the world epidemic: report of a WHO consultation.* Geneva: WHO

House of Commons Health Committee (2001) *Second report: public health: session 2000-1 HC30-I and HC30-II.* London: The Stationery Office

Summary: the brief was to look at how well the Trusts, Health Authorities and the Government were coordinated in delivering public health, looking in particular at agencies such as Health Action Zones, Health Improvement Programmes and Healthy Living Centres. As well as taking evidence, the Committee visited Cuba where good health outcomes are achieved and there is a high life expectancy in spite of poor resources and trade restrictions. Findings include:

- public health is underfunded and has a low profile
- the momentum gathered from *Saving lives (1997)* has largely dissipated: too much emphasis is placed on acute curative care, with waiting lists the only mark of effectiveness
- stronger leadership is needed and stronger partnerships for a broad-based approach to public health
- public health should be seen as an applied science, using knowledge to bring about change, not just gathering information for its own sake
- agencies should avoid constant reorganisation; consider creating incentives; build up the research base and learn from past experience
- Chief Medical Officer to publish long promised report as a matter of urgency

Further reading:

Department of Health (2001) *Government response to the House of Commons Select Committee on Health's second report on public health (cm5242).* London: HMSO

Hemmes, M. (1994) Cuba: its health care system may offer lessons for U.S. policy makers. *Hospitals and Health Networks* 68(9) 52-4

Hunter, David and Goodwin, Neil (2001) How to get promoted. *Health Service Journal* 111(5764) 26-7

Department of Health (2001) *The report of the Chief Medical Officer's project to strengthen the public health function.* London: Department of Health

Summary: long overdue report with extensive recommendations that include:

- improve public awareness, health surveillance and the evidence base
- improve coordination, establish a Public Health Forum and strengthen existing networks
- 'joined up working': share public health information and expertise at local and regional level; raise the profile of the Director of Public Health's annual report; promote flexible working between agencies
- promote sustainable community development with full public involvement
- public health workforce: to increase, to be multidisciplinary and adequately funded; within the workforce, strengthen leadership and proactive working and develop plans for education and training

Department of Health (2001) *National strategy for sexual health and HIV.* London: Department of Health

Summary: the variations in levels of sexual health services as well as an increase in the prevalence of sexually transmitted infections (STIs) have led to this strategy. The strategy is a ten-year commitment with fourteen proposals designed to raise the level of services and reduce the incidence of STIs, HIV and unwanted pregnancies. These proposals include:

- pilots of one-stop clinics
- primary care youth services
- screening for chlamydia and routine HIV testing in genitourinary medicine clinics
- ensuring parity in abortion services
- making contraceptive services available as well as hepatitis B vaccine

Chief Medical Officer (2002) *Getting ahead of the curve: a strategy for combating infectious diseases (including other aspects of health protection).* London: Department of Health

Summary: this fulfills one of the pledges of *Saving lives: our healthier nation (1999)* and takes in protection against chemical and radiological hazards. The present global situation: HIV/AIDS, malaria and T. B. account for millions of deaths each year, and experts agree that the threat of an influenza pandemic such as occurred after the First World War is not a question of 'whether', but 'when'. Risk of infection is increased by world travel, micro-organisms becoming more virulent and resistant to treatment, more people with compromised immunity and changes in the way we use land and the environment. In England, hospital-acquired infections may account for as many as 5,000 deaths while numbers diagnosed with HIV will rise to 29,000 by 2003. The document also notes the impact of crises due to BSE/vCJD, meningitis, influenza, bronchitis and e coli.

Causes: new diseases, animal-transmitted diseases, poor hygiene, below-standard medical practice and unpredictable situations such as the release of anthrax in the USA in 2001. Proposals include:

- to establish new agencies (especially since the abolition of local health authorities) for the surveillance, control and prevention of infectious diseases at national, regional and local levels - the National Infection Control Protection Agency, local health protection services and a national expert panel
- to improve systems of surveillance
- new action plans to establish priorities with: T. B., hospital-acquired infections, blood-borne and sexually transmitted diseases
- to appoint an Inspector of Microbiology along with an improved microbiology laboratory service
- to establish a plan to combat the threat of deliberate release of toxic agents
- improve public information, staff development and training, research and development and to review the law

Further reading:
Nicoll, A. and Murray, V. (2002) Health protection: a strategy and a national agency. *Public Health* 116(3) 129-37

O'Brien, M (2002) Health protection: the final straight? *Public Health* 116(3) 184-5

National Audit Office (2002) *Facing the challenge: NHS emergency planning in England: report by the Comptroller and Auditor General: HC36 session 2002-03*. London: The Stationery Office

Summary: although started before the terrorist attack on New York on 11th September 2001, this report was reviewed in the light of that event. The report finds the NHS in England ready to cope with the kinds of incidents we have already experienced such as train crashes. It views as unreasonable to expect the NHS to cope with disasters on a vast scale. At best, work has been very thorough on looking at assessment of risks and hazards and what is needed to cope with them. Recommendations include:

- incident planning and testing plans
- training personnel
- supply and provision of protective and decontamination equipment
- evening out geographical variation
- Department of Health to provide guidance and training for dealing with the release of hazardous substances
- chief executives of acute and ambulance trusts to identify any deficiencies in their major accident plans and ensure they include measures for dealing with mass casualties, chemical, biological, radiological and nuclear incidents

Chief Medical Officer (2003) *Winning ways: working together to reduce health associated infection in England*. London: Department of Health

Summary: findings include:

- infection during treatment and care is common with very expensive consequences
- the NHS in England does not perform well compared with the rest of Europe
- known, effective countermeasures are inconsistently implemented
- inadequate surveillance in the past, with not enough good information available to clinicians or patients
- hand washing is an essential activity but poor performance or irresponsibility not always the main barrier, in some settings there are poor facilities, no hand hygiene agents available, or no time

The report proposes improvements in seven 'action areas': 1) surveillance 2) reducing risk from invasive procedures 3) reducing reservoirs of infection 4) standards of hygiene 5) use of antibiotics 6) management and 7) research and development

Further reading:
Strachan-Bennett, S. (2003) Can nurses stop the rise of the hospital superbug? *Nursing Times* 100(1) 10-11

National Audit Office (2004) *Improving care by reducing the risk of hospital-acquired infection: a progress report: report by the Comptroller and Auditor General: HC876 session 2003-04.* London: The Stationery Office

Summary: the report looked at progress since 1999 and how countries in the rest of Europe deal with the issue. Whilst infection control has a higher priority, hospital-acquired infections have only slightly reduced because of conflicting pressures to pursue other policies and increased antibiotic resistance, with new strains of bacteria and viruses. The report also finds

- more staff education is needed to change behaviours
- inadequate information about the extent and costs of hospital acquired infection
- supports and endorses the Chief Medical Officer's report *Winning ways* with its seven areas of focus (see above)

Department of Health (2004) *Towards cleaner hospitals and lower rates of infection.* London: Department of Health

Summary: an action plan to improve standards of hygiene in hospitals, given that on the one hand cleanliness is a major concern for patients, on the other MRSA and other hospital-acquired infections are on the increase. The plan includes:

- measures to empower patients
- a charter for matrons
- independent inspections
- learning from the evidence and making best use of the latest research

Further reading:
Department of Health (2004) *A matron's charter: an action plan for cleaner hospitals.* London: Department of Health

NHS Estates (2001) *Housekeeping: a first guide to new, modern, dependable ward housekeeping services in the NHS.* London: Department of Health

Health Protection Agency Act 2004: chapter 17. London: The Stationery Office

Summary: first proposed in *Getting ahead of the curve (2002)*, the Act provides for a the Health Protection Agency Special Health Authority and the National Radiological Protection Board to be replaced by a single Health Protection Agency, with a view to dealing more effectively with epidemics of infectious diseases and the threat from chemical, biological, radiological and nuclear terrorism.

Further reading:
Dimond, B. (2004) The Health Protection Agency. *British Journal of Midwifery* 12(1) 20

Royal College of Physicians, Royal College of Paediatrics and Child Health and Faculty of Public Health Medicine (2004) *Storing up problems: the medical case for a slimmer nation.* London: Royal College of Physicians

Summary: the report is addressed to Government in education and health and also to the food industry and advertising. More than half the population is either overweight or obese; levels of obesity in children have risen from 5% to 9% in the 2-4 age group and from 5% to 16% in the 6-15 age group. Looks at the costs to the NHS and to international research that shows how obesity reduces life expectancy leading to cardiovascular disease, type 2 diabetes, stroke, cancer and osteoarthritis. Recommendations include:

- improved food labelling with incentives to promote sale of healthier foods
- education campaign with local initiatives to promote better eating and physical activity
- every NHS plan, policy and clinical care strategy to consider overweight and obesity with training given to health professionals
- more research needed to look at the causes of obesity, effective prevention and treatments

Further reading:

Nacif, A. P. (2004) Weighty matters: obesity takes hold. *Health Service Journal* 144(5895) 13 & 15

National Health and Medical Research Council (2003) *Overweight and obesity guidelines.* Sydney: National Health and Medical Research Council

House of Commons Health Committee (2004) *Obesity: third report of session 2003-04: HC 23-I.* London: The Stationery Office

Summary: reports similar findings to *Storing up problems (2004)* with obesity set to outstrip smoking as the chief cause of early death. Suggests today's children may be the first for whom life expectancy will fall. Estimates national costs of between £3.3 and £7.4 billion.
Causes:

- food: not just that we eat too much but what gets in the way of healthy eating such as: children have no cooking skills; instant meals are too easy to obtain; powerful advertising; 'unhealthy' food too attractively priced; food labelling is confusing
- exercise: the Department of Health set a target of 30 minutes exercise five times per week for but only one third of men and one quarter of women achieve this; the number of cars has doubled in 30 years where activities like walking and cycling have plummeted; children are increasingly sedentary; television viewing has doubled since the 1960s and all round physical activity has decreased through increased automation

Recommendations include:

- improve food labelling; prohibit advertising directed at children that undermines a parent's autonomy; food industry to alter pricing to make healthy foods more attractive
- more physical activity in schools; improve nutritional value of school meals

- condemns the Department of Transport for failing to produce its promised Walking Strategy, refers them to Danish town planning models that favour the walker and cyclist
- Government must resist anxiety of being called a 'nanny state', especially since they must pay the bill if nothing improves

Further reading:

Chief Medical Officer (2004) *At least five a week: evidence on the impact of physical activity and its relationship to health.* London: Department of Health

Department of Culture, Media and Sport and Strategy Unit (2002) *Game plan: a strategy for delivering the Government's sport and physical activity objectives.* London: Strategy Unit

Department of Transport (2003) *On the move: by foot: a discussion paper.* London: Department of Transport

Wanless, D. (2004) *Securing good health for the whole population.* London: HM Treasury

Summary: a second report from Derek Wanless that proposes a strategy for reducing preventable illness and improving public health. Points at the considerable difference in costs that would arise from people becoming responsible or 'fully engaged' with their own health. Notes however:

- the evidence-base is poor compared with regular medicine, with little evidence about the cost-effectiveness of public health measures and limited assessment of the impact of key polices to do with transport, agriculture etc
- previous target-setting has either been under or over-optimistic with poorly managed resources
- more careful monitoring is needed of the success of measures such as seat-belt wearing in cars or immunisation programmes
- whilst ultimately responsible for their health, individuals need more active support in making better decisions

The review makes 21 recommendations including:

- consider economic policies to promote health such as tax credits and/or taxing 'junk food'
- consistent national and local objectives to improve the health of the nation
- public health strategies and treatments should be monitored for their effectiveness and cost-effectiveness
- rather than focus on numbers of operations, health targets should look at health outcomes, comparing the benefits of preventing disease versus curing it
- consider how information and support might be better disseminated, via NHS Direct perhaps, with attempts to make health messages more understandable for those with poor literacy
- people should be regularly consulted about their understanding of major public health issues as well as the acceptability to them of possible state interventions
- major Government policies (e.g. road building or energy) should be assessed for their impact on health

- the NHS should work to improve the mental and physical health and wellbeing of its workforce

The review looks forward to the white paper *Choosing health (2004)*.

Further reading:
Edwards, N. (2003) Wanless in more. *Health Service Journal* 113(5880) 10-11

King's Fund, Health Development Agency and Department of Health (2004) *Public attitudes to public health policy.* London: King's Fund

Summary: public health has gained a higher profile since the latest Wanless report but while there is plenty of material looking at the public's attitude to the NHS, there is very little about what they think of health itself. This research paper looked into 1) health expectations 2) individual responsibility 3) the Government's role and 4) the NHS's role. Findings include:

- there is a class divide with people in higher socioeconomic groups enjoying and expecting better health
- the majority felt that individuals should take responsibility for their health and the health of their children, although more than 60% thought tackling poverty would have a greater impact on improving health than any public health measures. More than 40% - of whom most were in lower socioeconomic groups - thought that too many external factors stood in the way of good health
- Government should make the public aware of the price of poor health; providing information and advice and encouraging employers to promote health at work
- Government should prevent behaviours that put health at risk e.g. a ban on smoking, 'on street' drinking etc
- Government should provide healthy school meals and green spaces and educate the young about sexual health
- the NHS should provide information and support to prevent illness. Some respondents (in the higher socioeconomic groups) wanted this directed at people who are at risk, others (mostly lower socioeconomic groups) would prefer that help was directed at those who are already sick

Department of Health (2004) *Choosing health: making healthier choices easier (cm6374).* London: Department of Health

Summary: long-awaited white paper that follows: *Choosing health: a consultation on improving people's health (2004)*. Based on its findings this presents a new approach to public health. Rather than submit to heavy handed, top-down directives, people want access to good information and guidance that enables them to make free choices; they want support in lifestyle changes that is tailored to their needs and circumstances; they also want backup on all sides: from care services, national and local government, business, retailers and advertisers, the media, religious and voluntary organisations etc. Proposals include:

- smoking: by the end of 2008 all enclosed public and workplaces will be smoke free as well as all outlets preparing and serving food. There will tighter constraints on advertising and increased support for smokers who want to quit

- obesity and exercise: by mid 2005 all processed food to be labelled for fat, salt and sugar; Ofcom to invite companies to stop 'junk food' advertising aimed at children, with legislation in 2007 to force the change if necessary; NHS "trainers" to advise individuals about improving their health and fitness; initiatives for children and young people, encouraging exercise, healthier meals in schools, investment in school sport facilities etc; a task force to look at obesity

- sexual health: a national campaign against sexually transmitted infections and unplanned pregnancies; by 2008 all referrals to genitourinary clinics to have an appointment within 48 hours; Chlamydia screening in England by 2007

- alcohol: Ofcom to restrict adverts aimed at underage drinkers; investment to tackle problems at an early stage and cut down binge drinking

- mental health: tackle racial health inequalities; by the end of 2005 extend the *Sure Start* programmes; in 2005 offer guidelines for the management of mild to moderate mental health problems in the workplace

- initiatives for promoting health in the workplace, including for NHS staff

- funding for public health research

- a new Health Direct service to provide health information via telephone, internet and digital television

Further reading:

Coulter, A. and Rozansky, D. (2004) Full engagement in health: needs to begin in primary care. *British Medical Journal* 329(7476) 1197-1198

Muir Gray, J. A. (2003) *The resourceful patient.* Oxford: eRosetta

Supplementary reading:

Ballinger, Steve (2002) *Home sick: Shelter and Bradford & Bingley's campaign for healthy homes.* London: SHELTER

Department of Health (2001) *From vision to reality.* London: Department of Health

Department of Health (1998) *Health improvement programmes: planning for better health and better health care.* London: The Department of Health

Department of Health Standing Nursing and Midwifery Advisory Committee (1995) *Making it happen: public health: the contribution, role and development of nurses, midwives and health visitors: report of the Standing Nursing and Midwifery Advisory Committee.* London: HMSO

Department of Health *On the state of the public health: the annual report of the Chief Medical Officer of the Department of Health.* (annual) London: The Stationery Office

Department of Health and NHS Executive (1994) *Public health in England: roles and responsibilities of the Department of Health and the NHS.* London: HMSO

Gowman, N. and Coote, A. (2000) *Evidence and public health: towards a common framework.* London: King's Fund

Head, J. (2002) *Work environment, alcohol consumption and ill health: the Whitehall II study.* London: Health and Safety Executive

World Health Organisation (1998) *Social determinants of health: the solid facts.* Copenhagen: WHO

World Health Organisation (2004) *World report on knowledge for better health.* Geneva: WHO

4 Primary and Community Care

Audit Commission (1986) *Making a reality of community care.* London: HMSO

Summary: in spite of government policy to move away from long-term hospital care towards care in the community, the move is failing. While hospital care is being run down, community care is not keeping pace to fill the gap, especially in mental health; discrepancies are noted from one locality to another, again in mental health; the reduction in NHS hospitals has been met by an increase in private residential care, paid for by supplementary benefit at a cost of more than £500 million. The report's concern is that the money saved is being wasted and that some disabled and vulnerable people are missing out on care altogether. The following recommendations are offered:

- rationalise funding and issue short-term funds to cover the transition period
- social service and community care policies to be coordinated to allow cooperation between the various agencies and a multi-disciplinary team approach to an individual's care
- local responsibilities, authority and accountability to be clearly defined
- local authorities given greater power
- staff training to be given to prepare them for community care
- provision made for cost-effective voluntary organisations
- to do nothing is absolutely untenable: the assets released from the rundown of hospitals were inadequately redeployed and a 37% increase in the elderly population is projected over the next ten years

Further reading:
Trnobranski, P. H. (1995) Implementation of community care policy in the United Kingdom: will it be achieved? *Journal of Advanced Nursing* 21(5) 988-95

Department of Health (1988) *Community care: agenda for action.* (chair Roy Griffiths) London: HMSO

Summary: offers a plan for the care of adults in the community with a view to enabling individuals to receive the right care at the right time, to have a say and a choice in their care and where possible, to be cared for in their own homes. Proposals:

- appointing a Minister of State with responsibility for community care
- that local social services should assess/identify needs of individuals and locality; arrange for the delivery of care; design, organise and purchase non-health care services; all in collaboration with health authorities and voluntary and private providers
- that local social services should have responsibility for funding
- that central government should arrange for the transfer of funds and provide a significant proportion of the total cost

- that local authorities should have adequate management systems in place
- that health authorities should have continued responsibility for medical community health care services with GPs responsible for making local authorities aware of particular needs
- that local and health authorities should have the power to act jointly or as agents for each other
- that the functions of a community carer develop into a new occupation with appropriate training so that one person can provide whatever help is needed. For this to happen there needs to be an understanding about the contribution of other professionals in the field to avoid insularity

Further reading:
Rayner, M. (1990) Two steps ahead of Griffiths...community care. *Nursing Times* 86(15) 40-1

Shuttleworth, A. (1988) Whatever happened to the Griffiths Report? Community care. *Professional Nurse* 4(3) 119-20

Department of Health (1989) *Caring for people: community care in the next decade and beyond (cm849).* London: HMSO

Summary: endorses the recommendations of the Griffiths report and sets out six key objectives:

- to promote domiciliary, day care and respite services in order to enable people to live in their own homes
- practical support for carers to be a high priority
- the 'cornerstone' of community care to be a proper assessment of need and good case management
- to encourage the independent sector - voluntary and private
- to clarify the various caring agencies' responsibilities
- to establish a new funding structure with no incentive given in favour of residential and nursing home care

The report recognises the continuing need for long-term hospital care; that primary health care workers are generally a patient's first port of call and that the voluntary sector need a clear role with a sounder financial base to allow them a greater degree of certainty. Seven key changes are outlined:

- local authorities (LAs) to be responsible for assessing overall need, designing care arrangements and securing their delivery
- LAs to publish yearly plans for development
- LAs to make maximum use of the independent sector
- LAs to take responsibility for the financial support of people in residential and nursing homes
- applicants with no resources of their own to be eligible for the same levels of income support and housing benefit whether in their own or a nursing/residential home

- LAs to establish inspection and registration units to check on standards in their own and independent residential care homes
- a specific grant to be made available for the social care of the seriously mentally ill

Although the LAs are to take the lead responsibility, the report states that the Health Services must be responsible for maintaining good collaboration with Social Services and must contribute to the forming of the yearly community care plan.

Further reading:

Caring for people: community care. (1991) *Senior Nurse* 10(1) 1

NHS Management Executive (1993) *New world, new opportunities: report of a task group on nursing in primary health care.* London: HMSO

Wheeler, N. (1990) "Working for patients" and "Caring for people": the same philosophy? *British Journal of Occupational Therapy* 53(10) 409-14

Department of Health (1995) *Carers (Recognition and Services) Act 1995: chapter 12.* London: HMSO

Summary: this Act gives carers the right to request local authorities to assess their ability to provide adequate care and if necessary to provide additional resources to assist them in caring. The legislation formally recognises the care needs of disabled or elderly people at home, and the needs of their carers as well.

Further reading:

Andrews, J. (1995) Who cares for the carers? *Practice Nurse* 10(7) 450-1

George, M. (1995) Collaborative caring. *Nursing Standard* 9(46) 22-3

New act protects rights of carers. (1996) *Elderly Care* 8(3) 6

Department of Health (1996) *Choice and opportunity: primary care: the future (cm3390).* London: The Stationery Office

Summary: a white paper that proposes a need for legislation that will encourage local flexibility in organisation, staffing and finance in order to deliver primary care services appropriate to local needs and circumstances. The paper concentrates on GPs, dentists, pharmacists and optometrists. The paper proposes legislation that will enable those who wish it to pilot different types of contract, for the appointment of GPs.

Further reading:

Cole, A. (1996) Opportunity knocks. *Health Visitor* 69(12) 484-5

Department of Health (1996) *Primary care: delivering the future.* London: The Stationery Office

Summary: brings together themes raised in *Primary care: the future (1996)* and *The NHS: a service with ambitions (1996)*. Rather than radical change the paper proposes a direction for evolution towards a primary care-led NHS.

Aims and proposals:

- to enable local people to determine the service they want

- to coordinate all involved professionals: dentists, pharmacists, optometrists, social workers and housing officers as well as the primary health care team
- to improve professional development and knowledge-based decision-making
- to improve collaboration and cooperation so as to enable "seamless" management of care between organisations
- to improve the use of information technology
- patients to recognise their responsibility to the service as well as for their own health
- an increase in the proportion of government funding for primary care, including research and development funding
- practice staff to come in to the NHS Pension Scheme by September 1997
- to improve the range, quality and standard of work premises

Community Care (Direct Payments) Act 1996: chapter 30. London: The Stationery Office

Summary: provides for local authorities to make payments to individuals for them to buy care services direct, following a needs assessment.

National Health Service (Primary Care) Act 1997: chapter 46. London: The Stationery Office

Summary: builds on the last two white papers and legislates to give nurses and GPs the right to set up and run pilot schemes for providing primary care services.

Further reading:

Audit Commission (2003) *Transforming primary care: the role of primary care trusts in shaping and supporting general practice.* London: Audit Commission

General Practitioner's Committee (2004) *Personal medical services agreements: guidance for GPs.* London: British Medical Association

Thomas, S. (1997) Developing the primary care led NHS. *Journal of Community Nursing* 11(6) 8-11

Audit Commission (1998) *Home alone: the role of housing in community care.* London: Audit Commission

Summary: a first document to point out the vital role played by housing services in the delivery of community care. The work of housing agencies includes: provision of social housing, adapting properties, provision of support for vulnerable clients, coordinating efforts with social services. There are four chapters:

1. Housing Services comprise alarms and adaptations; sheltered housing or with personal support for people with disabilities; resettling the homeless and offering support to enable people to remain, coping in their own homes. Housing amounts to a lower level of support but serves a huge population, in greater numbers than health or social services. Their finance comes from central government, local housing departments, health authorities and social services, housing corporations

and RSL. A crisis is emerging because with an increasing demand for the service, the stock of social housing has gone down, the role of housing authorities is changing and major changes in housing benefit are imminent.

2. Effective delivery is failing because of poor collaboration with health authorities and social services; inadequate identification of needs and poor planning: failure to intervene early enough is leading to a reactive approach to crises and delays.

3. Local level solutions would include: a system for gathering information about local needs; reviewing performance; awareness of provision and better use of resources.

4. At a national level: the funding regime needs overhauling: costs are shunted and there is poor information about the actual cost of services. Uncoordinated policies, e.g. the impact of closure of long-stay psychiatric facilities, lead to major problems in service delivery, and it is not clear 'who owns the problems'.

Further reading:

Watson, Lynn (1998) *High hopes: making housing and community care work.* London: Joseph Rowntree Foundation

Henwood, Melanie (1998) *Ignored and invisible? Carers' experience of the NHS: report of a UK research survey commissioned by the Carers National Association.* London: Carers National Association

Summary: the report gives the context of health policy under the Labour government followed by a profile of the 3,000 respondents to the survey. Subsequent sections examine:

*   provision of support: most are caring alone with limited support from social services, district nursing and other home services such as chiropody. Those who received no support believed support would have been helpful
*   many carers have health problems of their own, reporting physical injury and treatment for stress-related illness as the result of caring
*   provision of information is inadequate and often has to be pushed for
*   hospital discharge and after care arrangements are often poor
*   NHS staff: GPs were rated highest, followed by district nurses; hospital social workers were not highly rated
*   the top priorities for carers were: funding, cooperation between health and social services, the need for GPs to continue to make home visits and for all health staff to be trained in awareness of carers' needs

The chief recommendations are that pressure should be brought to bear on the NHS to meet the requirements of the *Carers (Recognition and Services) Act 1995* and on the Department of Health to take responsibility for improving the coherence of health and social care services.

Further reading:

Rowlands, Olwen (1998) *Informal carers: an independent study carried out by the Office for National Statistics on behalf of the Department of Health as part of the 1995 general household survey.* London: The Stationery Office

Department of Health (1998) *Modernising social services: promoting independence, improving protection, raising standards (cm4169).* London: The Stationery Office

Summary: long awaited reform that begins by noting six stumbling blocks to effective social care:

- protection: inadequate safeguards exist to protect the vulnerable
- coordination: conflict between authorities about who is to pay for what care
- inflexibility: help should be needs-led, not just what the service can offer
- role: clients don't know what help they can get from whom and to what standard
- inconsistency: uneven levels of service across the country
- inefficiency: great variations in cost from council to council

The plan for improvement includes:

- adults: direct payments to people over 65 should support their need for independent living and give real control over provision of service. Social services to have nationally established objectives and priorities, regulating who gets what and conducting satisfaction surveys
- children: tougher inspection arrangements for their protection; funding for the Quality Protects programme to improve children's social services; improved educational opportunities for children in care as well as help with the transition to adulthood
- protection: new systems for protecting vulnerable children and adults including eight regional 'Commissions for Care Standards'
- standards: a social care training strategy and the establishment of a GSCC - General Social Care Council - to set ethical standards and standards of practice
- partnerships with health: pooling budgets, improving partnerships with housing and other services
- improving delivery and efficiency: local authorities to be set targets, published annually, for quality and efficiency. Where standards are not met, central government to take action

Further reading:

Department of Health (1998) *Partnership in action: new opportunities for joint working between health and social services: a discussion document.* London: Department of Health

Douglas, Anthony (1998) Motherhood and apple pie. *Community Care* 3.12.1998 12

Philpot, Terry (1998) Let history judge. *Community Care* 3.12.1998 18-20

Social Exclusion Unit (1998) *Bringing Britain together: a national strategy for neighbourhood renewal (cm4045).* London: The Stationery Office

Summary: begins by describing how Britain has become a divided country with the poorest neighbourhoods locked into a downward spiral, becoming more rundown and more prone to social problems and unemployment. The strategy for renewal is based on investment in people and involving the whole community to provide solutions.

The plan includes:

- tackling unemployment
- good housing and neighbourhood management
- the Sure Start programme, improving prospects for young people
- improving access to basic services such as banks and shops

The strategy is to be coordinated by the Social Exclusion Unit for England and equivalent agencies for Wales, Scotland and Northern Ireland.

Further reading:

Alcock, P. (1998) Bringing Britain together? *Community Care* 26.11.1998 18-24

Rehal, F. and Langley, H. (2004) Ensuring a Sure Start. *Community Practitioner* 77(5) 168-71

Rosser, J. (2002) Sure Start midwifery: the reality of making practice relevant to health needs. *MIDIRS Midwifery Digest* 12(1) 18-20

Department of Social Security (1999) *Opportunity for all: tackling poverty and social exclusion (cm4445).* London: The Stationery Office

Summary: a white paper that outlines the extent of poverty and social exclusion in the UK and then describes a strategy to tackle the problem in four sections:

- children and young people
- people of working age
- older people
- communities

Based on three principles: *prevention* - tackling causes; *creating opportunity* and *empowerment* - investing in individuals, the strategy is to be long-term, flexible and collaborative. Recommendations include:

- investment in early years, education and help for families
- reducing teenage pregnancy
- helping people into employment, creating employment zones to improve opportunities in the poorest areas
- lifelong learning
- equal opportunities for the disabled and older people
- pension reform
- tackling crime
- improving access to services including cultural and leisure
- a National Strategy for Neighbourhood Renewal
- Information Technology Learning Centres

Further reading:

Geddes, Mike (2000) Social exclusion - new language, new challenges for local authorities. *Public Money and Management* 20(2) 55-60

Reeves, R. and Wintour, P. (1999) The poverty gap: help the poor? Well we'll have to find them first. *The Observer* 19.9.99 18

Department of Health (1999) *Caring about carers: a national strategy for carers.* London: H.M. Government

Summary:

- one in eight people are informal carers
- 855,000 of these care for more than 50 hours per week
- three fifths receive no visitor support services
- arrangements for meeting their needs are inconsistent and patchy

To improve the lives of informal carers, the paper outlines a package of measures that include:

- improved access to information and a charter outlining standards of service in long-term care
- improving carer involvement in service planning and provision
- protecting carers so that they can work and take breaks
- financial measures such as a second pension for carers; reducing council tax for disabled people; support for neighbourhood services

The document includes a chapter on the protection of young carers and appendixes with helplines and a code of good practice for service providers.

Further reading:

Nolan, Mike (1999) National strategy for carers: the way forward? *British Journal of Nursing* 8(4) 194

Care Standards Act 2000: chapter 14. London: The Stationery Office

Summary: this Act comes into force in April 2002 and pulls together proposals and recommendations for social services in England and Wales taken from recent reports such as *Modernising social services (1998)*. The aim is to regulate:

- children's homes
- care homes
- residential family centres
- independent hospitals and clinics
- nurse agencies
- independent medical agencies
- voluntary adoption agencies

The key provisions include:

- setting up a National Care Standards Commission (with equivalent bodies in Wales, Scotland and Northern Ireland), to regulate care and care homes, children's homes and other independent, private and voluntary agencies
- social care workers (defined as "a person engaged in the provision of personal care for any person") to register with new independent Councils such as the GSCC (and equivalent bodies in Wales, Scotland and Northern Ireland see *Accountable care: the new GSCC (1999)*). These will also regulate the training and education of social workers and set standards for social work using codes of conduct and practice amongst other things

- reforms the regulation of child minding and day care provision, transferring responsibility from local authorities to a new arm of Ofsted. New, national standards will require those wishing to work or come into contact with older children will have to demonstrate their suitability to do so
- Secretary of State to maintain a list of those considered unsuitable for work with vulnerable adults, the list to operate in a similar way to that established under the *Protection of Children Act 1999: chapter 14*

Further reading:
Nazarko, L. (2001) A new broom: the Care Standards Act. *Nursing Management* 7(8) 6-9

O'Neale, V. (2000) *Excellence not excuses: inspection of services for ethnic minority children and families.* London: The Stationery Office

Summary: published in the wake of the Stephen Lawrence inquiry, this report looks into issues significant to ethnic minority families, and aims to help local councils improve their awareness and improve their services to such families. The report recognises that personal and institutional racism, immigration, separated families and nationality laws can create particular problems for ethnic minorities. It finds that although intentions are good, most local councils do not have appropriate strategies for delivering quality services (although there are exceptions) and such services that are offered are not sensitive to the needs of ethnic minorities. In addition the report finds that not enough consideration is given to equal opportunities and the specific needs and problems of ethnic minority staff working in social services.

Further reading:
Home Office (1999) *The Stephen Lawrence Inquiry (cm4262-I).* (chair William Macpherson) London: The Stationery Office

Gordon, David et al (2000) *Poverty and social exclusion in Britain.* London: Joseph Rowntree Foundation

Summary: this report represents the first findings of the most comprehensive study of poverty in this country. Poverty is measured in terms of 'deprivation from goods, services and activities which the majority ... defines as being ... necessities'. It also considers ways of measuring social exclusion. The report begins by noting the Government's commitment to ending poverty - child poverty in 20 years - and in the subsequent chapters looks at: adult poverty, child poverty and the growth of poverty and social exclusion. Lack of paid work as well as insufficient child benefit and dependency allowances are seen as the chief causes of poverty and social exclusion with poverty at the root of the majority of social problems.

Further reading:
Benn, Melissa (2000) It just can't be done. *Community Care* 12.10.2000 14

Brittain, Samuel (2000) The poor need not always be with us. *Search* (33) 8-11

Frean, A. (2000) Quarter of households now living in poverty. *The Times* 11.9.2000 10

Green, Roger (2000) Applying a community needs profiling approach to tackling service user poverty. *British Journal of Social Work* 30(3) 287-303

Maltby, Tony and Walker, Alan (1997) Poverty and social exclusion. *Working with Older People* 1(2) 11-15

Norton, Cherry (2000) One-sixth of Britain's children living below the poverty line. *Independent* 11.9.2000

Office for National Statistics (2000) *Social inequalities 2000 edition.* London: The Stationery Office

Summary: an official report that looks at poverty and for the first time, social exclusion. The difficulties defining terms are discussed: poverty being described in 'relation to average standards of living' and social exclusion encompassing 'notions of participation in society'. The data is based on snapshots of the population with some information relating to change in society. There is data on four main headings:

- people and places: population growth and distribution, age and ethnic status. Information about mortgages, housing and car ownership are related to social status
- income and wealth: distribution of wealth according to age, social and ethnic status, gender and lone parenthood
- education, training and skills: gender differences in educational achievement; the relationship between jobs and skills requirements
- work: this looks at full and part-time work, noting gender, age and ethnic differences

Further reading:
Travis, Alan (2000) How gap between rich and poor has grown. *The Guardian* 11.5.2000 8

Audit Commission (2001) *Change here!: managing change to improve local services.* London: Audit Commission

Summary: this is aimed at all public service managers in the light of all the reforms instigated by the Labour Government since coming to office in 1997. For change to be 'owned', the guide emphasises the need for all change programmes to be user/client focused and tailored to local circumstances. The responsibilities for Government, service staff and in particular, service leaders are indicated and there is a discussion of the various merits of four types of organisational change namely: *surgery* and *transformation* ('step' changes) and *operational gains* and *evolutionary learning* ('incremental' changes).

Further reading:
Iles, Valerie and Sutherland, Kim 'Organisational change: a review for healthcare managers, professionals and researchers.' [WWW]
http://www.lshtm.ac.uk/php/hsru/sdo/whatsnew.htm (11.02.02)

Henwood, Melanie (2001) *Future imperfect? Report of the King's Fund Care and Support Inquiry.* London: King's Fund

Summary: the Inquiry was set up to examine care and support for the 2 million adults in Britain needing care. The method involved taking written submissions, holding discussions and consultative meetings with service users and carers. On the one hand the Inquiry found a commitment to providing a quality service, with many examples of good practice. On the other hand, inadequate funding and bearing the brunt of negative criticism has lead to low morale. Directed at the GSCC, the Department of Health, the Department of Education and Training, trusts, the Learning and Skills Council and local authorities, the Inquiry's recommendations arise from the following issues:

- a conflict between promoting quality and not enough funding, even to keep the service 'standing still'
- underdeveloped skills and knowledge from a traditionally unskilled workforce
- problems with recruitment and retention
- inconsistent regulation and staff training
- inadequate management
- the need to involve clients and their carers when receiving and planning services
- historically the care sector suffers from poor image and low status

Jarvis, Sarah (2001) *Skill mix in primary care: implications for the future.* London: Department of Health, Medical Practices Committee

Summary: in spite of an increase in the use of skill mix there is a lack of evidence that skill mix is cost effective, safe or satisfactory for users and providers. The report summarises some of the existing evidence on skill mix e.g.: in some areas of nursing, skill mix has led to deskilling and reduced morale among staff. The new NHS Workforce Development Confederations have the remit to review workforce development plans in the health economy

Coe, A. (2002) *Modernising services to transform care: inspection of how councils are managing the modernisation agenda in social care.* London: Department of Health

Summary: the result of inspections of local councils made in the light of recommendations outlined in *Modernising social services (1998).* Reasons for councils' success include:

- setting out and owning a clear vision at councillor / senior manager level
- effective communication between all staff
- turning visions into effective business plans and strategies
- staff feeling supported and clear about what they have to do
- effective recruitment and retention of staff

Community Care (Delayed Discharges) Act 2003: chapter 5. London: The Stationery Office

Summary: Delivering the NHS plan (2002) wanted to reduce the number of 'bed blockers': patients waiting and safe to go home from hospital but prevented from doing so because of local authorities' failure to provide a continuing care package. The Act is meant as an incentive to local authorities to assess needs and plan services either before admission - in the case of elective surgery - or between admission and discharge. The Act imposes a fine on local authorities, payable to the healthcare provider for every day that discharge is delayed. In certain circumstances local authorities are prevented from charging for community care and carer's services.

Further reading:
Lymbery, M. and Millward, A. (2004) Delayed discharge: preparing for reimbursement. *Journal of Integrated Care* 12(4) 28-34

NHS Confederation (2003) *The new general medical services contract: investing in general practice.* London: British Medical Association and NHS Confederation

Summary: points include:

- GPs to have greater flexibility about the services they offer over and above the core service
- incentives for delivering evidence-based care that improves patient experience
- modernisation that includes improving premises and developing I.T.
- support for GPs in deprived or remote areas and for themselves to achieve a 'healthy balance' between work and personal life
- transparent, equitable payment for practices
- promote patient empowerment and broaden the range of high quality services
- simplify the regulation of how a contract is worked out

Further reading:
Department of Health (2003) *Investing in general practice: the new general medical services contract.* London: Department of Health

The National Health Service (General Medical Services Contracts) Regulations 2004. London: The Stationery Office

Barnes, J. and Gurney, G. (2004) *Performance action teams: supporting improvement in social care services.* London: Department of Health

Summary: Performance Action Teams were introduced in 2002 to improve performance of councils. The report summarises how bringing in external assistance helped councils to their social services and notes the key points for success including:

- need all participants to engage willingly in the activities
- there should be clear goals and shared agreement
- councils should show consistently good management and leadership
- PATs had most credibility when they had a wide range of skills and used people who had social services experience
- the most successful PATs involved the councils at every stage of work

Carers (Equal Opportunities) Act 2004: chapter 15. London: The Stationery Office

Summary: develops the *Carers (Recognition and Services) Act 1995* and the *Carers and Disabled Children Act 2000* providing as follows:

- requires local authorities to tell carers they may be entitled to an assessment
- part of that assessment must take into account whether the carer is working or in education or undertaking 'leisure activities' or who wishes to do any of these things
- sets a formal basis for cooperation between local authorities and other agencies

Supplementary Reading

Audit Commission (1999) *First assessment: a review of district nursing services in England and Wales.* London: Audit Commission

Audit Commission (2002) *Homelessness: responding to the new agenda.* London: Audit Commission

Audit Commission (2004) *Making an impact: minimising bureaucracy, maximising impact on public services.* London: Audit Commission

Banks, P. and Roberts, E. (2001) *More breaks for carers?* London: King's Fund

Brooks, Fiona and Gillam, Stephen (2001) *New beginnings - why patient and public involvement in primary care?* London: King's Fund

Carers National Association (1999) *Taking action to support carers.* London: King's Fund

Department of Health (1998) *The new NHS: modern dependable: primary care groups; delivering the agenda.* London: Department of Health

DHSS (1986) *Neighbourhood nursing: a focus for care.* (chair Julia Cumberlege) London: HMSO

Family Policy Studies Centre (2000) *Family poverty and social exclusion.* London: FPSC

Farrell, Christine et al (1999) *A new era for community care? What people want from health, housing and social care services.* London: King's Fund

Harrison, Anthony (ed) *Health care UK: an annual review of health care policy.* (annual) London: King's Fund

Henwood, Melanie (2001) *Future imperfect? Report of the King's Fund Care and Support Inquiry.* London: King's Fund

Holzhausen, Emily Pearlman, Vicky and Jackson, Annie (2001) *Caring on the breadline: the financial implications of caring.* London: Carers National Association

Homelessness Act 2000: chapter 7. London: The Stationery Office

Howarth, Catherine and Kenway, Peter (1998) *Monitoring poverty and social exclusion: why Britain needs a key indicators report.* London: New Policy Institute

Kohner, Nancy and Hill, Alison P. (2000) *Help! Does my patient know more than me?* London: King's Fund

Lucas, K. Grosvenor, T. and Simpson, R. (2001) *Transport, the environment and social exclusion.* London: York Publishing Services for Joseph Rowntree

National Audit Office (2004) *Reforming NHS dentistry: ensuring effective management of risks*. London: The Stationery Office

NHS Executive (1996) *Primary care: the future.* London: NHS Executive

O'Neale, V. (2000) *Excellence not excuses: inspection of services for ethnic minority children and families.* London: The Stationery Office

Warner, L. and Wexler, S. (1998) *Eight hours a day and taken for granted.* London: Princess Royal Trust for Carers

5 Older People

Henwood, Melanie (1992) *Through a glass darkly: community care and elderly people.* London: King's Fund

Summary: a critique of community care of the elderly following the white paper *Caring for people (1989).* Considers:

- demographic changes
- the shift in policy from direct care to home care and support for informal carers
- poor interaction between health and social care provision at all levels
- demand for residential care.

Recommends a clarification of the role of the NHS and responsibilities of the health authorities and development of NHS nursing homes, their providing an excellent model for continuing care.

Neill, June and Williams, Jenny (1992) *Leaving hospital: elderly people and their discharge to community care: report to the Department of Health.* London: HMSO

Summary: small sample research by the National Institute of Social Work Research Unit that set out to describe hospital discharge in terms of organisation of services, assessment of clients, roles of home care workers and to evaluate the effectiveness of discharge services in terms of relevance and impact on the client.

More elderly people are being discharged from hospital quicker and sicker and yet:

- no policies have been written to react to this development
- with scarce resources, conflict has increased amongst managers as well as between health authorities and social services. There is also poor communication between primary and secondary care agencies
- rehabilitation facilities are rare
- although half the local authorities examined had some kind of discharge scheme, even where there was good practice, finance could not be relied on to continue

Recommendations:

- authorities to have written hospital discharge schemes with a single appointed organiser and stable financing
- planning for discharge should begin as soon as possible after admission
- there should be early reassessment soon after discharge
- there should be an established minimum standard of home help to include housework

Department of Health (1996) *A new partnership for care in old age (cm3242).* London: HMSO

Summary: in view of the present cost to individuals of long term care (as much as £20,000) this consultation paper proposes a partnership between individual and state to provide for long term care in old age. The Government has to:

- promote awareness of what a person needing care might face by way of means testing and the cost to themselves
- encourage individuals to make their own provision for care
- encourage the finance industry to offer services that will allow for the provision of care

Audit Commission (1997) *The coming of age: improving care services for older people.* London: Audit Commission

Summary: a report following two studies in continuing care and commissioning community care. The first half of the report concerns assessing and arranging care. The recommendations are:

- health authorities and social services to agree on their respective responsibilities
- there should be a coordinated approach to assessment
- discharge delays to be audited and an individual appointed to monitor process
- time standards to be agreed in fulfilling a care arrangement
- clients and their carers to be kept better informed and involved by social services
- home care services to be reviewed regularly by social services
- care managers to be given greater power and financial control

All of these are considered urgent, short-term actions.

The other half of the report concerns 'rebalancing' services so that care is delivered appropriately:

- health authorities and social services to 'map' what services are available to them and review what services are really needed
- mapping and review processes to be backed up by an information package that will allow for easy updating
- health authorities and trusts to consider ways of reducing hospital admissions and improving rehabilitation
- social services to improve relations with the independent sector
- social services to develop financial mechanisms and consider ways of rewarding good practice
- social services to develop more 'watertight' monitoring processes

All of these are considered 'medium term' actions. Three further Audit Commission reports in 2000 look at particular aspects of elderly care, see below.

Further reading:
Littlechild, Rosemary, and Glasby, Jon (2001) Emergency hospital admissions: older people's perceptions. *Education and Ageing* 16(1) 77-90

Clinical Standards Advisory Group (1998) *Community health care for elderly people.* (chair June Clark) London: Stationery Office

Summary: a commissioned report involving visits to sample NHS trusts, interviews with providers and users of services as well as carers; and a prospective study of a small sample of patients following their discharge from hospital.

Main findings:

- great variability in range, level and quality of service
- gaps in the provision of service including physiotherapy, rehabilitation, respite care and equipment
- poorly managed hospital discharge
- poor coordination and understanding between health and social services
- inappropriate use of private care in nursing and residential care homes
- problems with process and outcomes of contracting for community health services

Recommendations:

- there should be published minimum standards of provision
- skill mix of community staff to be reviewed and local criteria published for availability of and eligibility for services
- greater effort to improve discharge procedures, fulfilling existing policies where these are deemed adequate
- based on categories of need, distinctions between health and social care to be clearly defined
- nursing care to be NHS funded in preference to saving money using private services. Private care as a whole subject to greater regulation; the *Registration of Homes Act 1984* to be reviewed
- drawn up in consultation with the professionals who deliver the service, there should be longer-term, "clinically relevant" contracts for community health services

Further reading:
Newton, John (1998) The muddle of community health care for the elderly. *British Journal of Community Health Nursing* 3(2) 60

Clark, Heather Dyer, Sue and Horwood, Jo (1998) *That bit of help: the high value of low level preventative services for older people.* Bristol: The Policy Press and London: Joseph Rowntree Foundation

Summary: the report of a study that assessed the value of low level helping services. These amount to help with gardening, laundry and about the house. The participants in the study see these services as 'help' not 'care' and as vital in letting them remain at home and out of expensive residential care. The continuing relationship with the helper is also important. The report dislikes the distinction between the value put upon 'high level' personal care and 'low level' domestic help and challenges the low priority given to the 'unskilled' help since participants - especially older women - showed a consistently high regard for the skills involved. Recommendations include:

- policy makes and service providers to look beyond the short term and reconsider the value of 'low level' help
- monies for these services might be ring-fenced
- a tool is needed to measure cost-effectiveness and prove the worth of preventive strategies

Further reading:
Clark, H. (1998) Keeping the house up. *Community Care* 16.7.1998 22-23

Health Advisory Service 2000 (1999) *Not because they are old: an independent inquiry into the care of older people on acute wards in general hospitals.* London: Department of Health

Summary: results of an inquiry, listing a catalogue of shortcomings in the acute care of the elderly. These include:
- long periods of waiting in discomfort
- neglected ward environments and a lack of basic supplies
- staff shortages and heavy work loads leading to poor communication and failure to respect privacy and dignity
- problems with food, feeding and nutrition
- problems with discharge planning and care

Recommendations include:
- full involvement in planning of care
- combating the negative attitude that associates old age with ill health
- prejudices and marginalisation of older people to be tackled in terms of range and quality of services
- role of ward manager to be promoted and safe staffing levels and skill mix to be assured
- named individual responsible for feeding and nutrition
- access to specialist knowledge assured twenty four hours a day, seven days a week
- promotion of a National Service Framework for Older People to determine standards of care

Royal Commission on Long Term Care (1999) *With respect to old age: long term care - rights and responsibilities (cm4192).* (chair Stewart Sutherland) London: The Stationery Office

Summary: current provision for long-term care cares for the poorest whilst impoverishing those with medium assets and driving many into residential care when this may not be the best option. On the principle that paying for care should be fair and shared between state and individual the report recommends:
- costs should be split between personal care and the costs of housing and living. Personal care to be assessed and determined according to need and covered by general taxation. Housing and living costs to be subject to a means-determined co-payment based on a person's income and savings

- a National Care Commission should be established to monitor and advise on trends and developments

The report dismisses long term care pensions schemes as putting an unfair burden on the young and also notes: the role of housing will become increasingly important; there should be support for informal carers, and the role of advocacy should be developed.

Further reading:

The other agenda (editorial) (1999) *Community Care* 4.3.1999 15

Mangan, Paul (1999) With respect to old age. *British Journal of Community Health Nursing* 4(4) 160

Kohler, Mervyn (1999) Organising the long term care of elderly people. *British Journal of Nursing* 8(3) 129

Department of Health (2000) *The NHS plan: the Government's response to the Royal Commission on Long Term Care (cm4818-II).* London: The Stationery Office

Summary: the Government broadly accepts the Commission's recommendations outlined in *With respect to old age (1999)*. The chief exceptions are that the Government sees no need to establish the cost of supporting residential care, and whilst nursing care in care homes is to be free, personal care is not.

Further reading:

Anon (2000) Blow to elderly care, say nurses. *Nursing Times* 96(31) 7

Audit Commission (2000) *Fully equipped: the provision of equipment to older or disabled people in England and Wales.* London: Audit Commission

Summary: this report starts with the premise that efficient equipment services promote independence and improve quality of life. It looks at whether the service is providing value for money and whether it is effective in giving independence to users. The report finds that provision varies widely and does not relate well to demand. Problems include poor quality of equipment, small fragmented services without leadership or management and poor cost-effectiveness when service processes do not meet users' initial needs and have to be repeated. Recommendations:

- local health authorities to have a central specialist service for complex problems and should provide support and leadership to local, less specialised services
- National Priorities Guidance should include these services
- standards of good practice should be established by users, professionals and suppliers
- trust managers to establish quality improvement plans for those equipment service providers that have been identified as substandard by user surveys, local audits or management reviews

Audit Commission (2000) *Forget me not: mental health services for older people.* London: Audit Commission

Summary: this is another of the series of reports promoting the independence of older people. (see *The coming of age - 1997*) The six chapters cover:

- the nature of mental health problems in old age
- how people get access to services and how to support carers and service providers
- the range of services available in the community
- the range of services available in hospital and residential care
- the need for good communication and coordination between the agencies using the Care Programme Approach
- the need for strategic planning

For the first time, auditors have been appointed to audit mental health services for older people in England and Wales.

Further reading:
Benbow, Susan M. and Lennon, Sean P. (2000) Forget me not: mental health services for older people. *Psychiatric Bulletin* 24(11) 403-4

Audit Commission (2000) *The way to go home: rehabilitation and remedial services for older people.* London: Audit Commission

Summary: another in the series of reports promoting independence for older people. Rehabilitation provision is not consistent or reliable in this country, even though it promotes independence and lessens unnecessary admissions to nursing and residential homes. The report defines the nature and scope of rehabilitation and gives examples of good practice in acute, intermediate and community-based service. The recommendations include:

- trusts to set up and/or develop stroke units
- acute, intermediate and community-based services to be coordinated with a care pathway approach
- need good multidisciplinary teamworking with effective communication especially at times of transfer
- trusts to develop screening and assessment services
- good workforce planning and development
- close involvement of health and social care services with geriatricians
- financial flexibility to enable new initiatives

Deeming, Chris (2001) *A fair deal for older people? Public views on the funding of long-term care.* London: King's Fund

Summary: the result of a public opinion poll following the *NHS plan: the Government's response to the Royal Commission on Long Term Care (2000).* There was wide support for the Government's decision to offer free nursing care but most did not agree with means-testing those people who need personal care. Wealthier respondents were in the majority among those willing to pay.

Department of Health (2001) *National service framework for older people.* London: Department of Health

Summary: following *A first class service: quality in the new NHS (1998)* this detailed document sets eight standards for the health and social care of older people. Each standard outlines an aim, a definition and a standard rationale with key interventions and a timescale for completion. The eight standards cover:

1. age discrimination
2. person-centred care
3. intermediate care: bridging the gap between acute and primary services
4. general hospital care
5. stroke
6. falls
7. mental health
8. health promotion

A separate document covers the medicines-related aspects of the NSF. Guidelines are offered for local implementation and national support.

Further reading:

Age Concern England (2001) *Age Concern's response to the NSF for older people.* London: Age Concern England

Black, D. (2001) NSF preview. *Geriatric Medicine* 30(1) 11-4

Davies, C. (2001) Nursing blueprint for elderly care. *Nursing Times* 97(9) 24-6

Department of Health (2001) *Medicines and older people: implementing medicines-related aspects of the NSF for older people.* London: Department of Health

Lothian, Kate and Philip, Ian (2001) Maintaining the dignity and autonomy of older people in the healthcare setting. *British Medical Journal* 322(7287) 668-70

Wellard, Sarah (2001) Framework marks assault on age discrimination. *Community Care* 5.4.2001 10-11

Audit Commission (2002) *Fully equipped: assisting independence.* London: Audit Commission

Summary: since the Commission's first report in 2000, the following improvements are noted:

- introduction of hearing screening for neonates
- improved availability of digital hearing aids
- the Government plan to improve and integrate equipment services in the community

However many problems remain the same:

- long delays before receiving equipment
- over stringent exclusion criteria
- up to 6 years waiting for equipment
- despondency among service managers
- poor integration of mobility services

Overall the service is not found to be needs-led, nor integrated with the rest of health and social care services and there is ineffectual commissioning in spite of proven worth of equipment services to keep people "on their feet" and away from readmission to hospitals.

Roberts, E. Robinson J. and Symour, L. (2002) *Old habits die hard: tackling age discrimination in health and social care.* London: King's Fund

Summary: the result of a confidential telephone survey of health and social service managers in England. The report finds that ageism is endemic, difficult to identify and whilst most managers are responding positively to the *National Service Framework for Older People (2001)* the timeframe is tight with resources and support inadequate. Social services are traditionally organised by age group, with older people given fewer choices and a more basic level of care. On the other hand expectations are lower: on the whole older people and their families are reluctant to complain about their care. Recommendations include:

- make clear the meaning and consequences of ageism
- develop benchmarking
- develop education and training for staff
- legislate to outlaw age discrimination in health and social care
- examine national social policies in order to rule out ageism

Further reading:
Scott, H. (2000) Age discrimination should be outlawed in the NHS. *British Journal of Nursing* 9(1) 4

Tonks, A. (1999) Medicine must change to serve an ageing society: eradicate age discrimination and increase resources. *British Medical Journal* 319(7223) 1450-1

Age Discrimination (no.2) Bill. (2002) London: The Stationery Office

Summary: this would make it unlawful to discriminate against someone on the grounds of age, with regards to employment and providing goods and services. The Bill provides for an Age Equality Commission and outlines its activities. It would place a duty on public bodies to promote age equality in employment practices and in providing services and would make it unlawful for employers to set a retirement age in work contracts.

Carrier, J. (2003) *Integrated services for older people: building a whole system approach in England.* London: Audit Commission

Summary: proposes a strategy for joint agency working for streamlined care, thus promoting independence and avoiding the common experience where help is given but only in part, where information is patchy and confused and only ever reacting to crisis. The report highlights the good health of older people with only about 14% using care services at any one time, and it stresses the need for services to look at the 86% and promote their need for independence. The system can work when it is focused on users and where agencies recognise their interdependence, their shared goals and their need for good communication. Qualities needed for an effective system include leadership, teamwork, good information and a single coordinated assessment process.

Commission for Health Improvement (2003) *Emerging themes: services for older people.* London: Commission for Health Improvement

Summary: based on a detailed examination of older people, stroke, and fractured neck of femur (FNOF) in 17 reviews published between August 2002 and February 2003 and also a review of actions that CHI had asked trusts to take concerning those three areas. Issues for concern include:

- privacy and treating patients with respect
- variations in access to specialist stroke services; some environments not suitable for stroke rehabilitation; in some trusts dedicated stroke teams and facilities are not in place
- staff shortages in all areas and professions
- elderly care not coordinated between the various agencies
- delays for FNOF surgery caused by elective surgery and surgical emergencies taking priority

Examples of good practice include:

- some organisations have involved users in delivery and planning of stroke services
- services have improved as the result of acting on audit findings
- in some areas stroke services are provided by multidisciplinary teams
- organisations are using the *NSF for Older People (2001)* to guide their care

National Audit Office (2003) *Ensuring the effective discharge of older patients from NHS acute hospitals: report by the Comptroller and Auditor General: HC392: session 2002-3.* London: The Stationery Office

Summary: although the majority of older patients are discharged when fit, an estimate in 2002 showed that about 9% were delayed, i.e. still occupying beds. This is not good for the patients concerned and is costly to the NHS when a bed is needed for someone else. The report looks at three areas in particular:

1. efficiency of acute hospitals at handling discharge
2. effectiveness of their liaison with other primary care agencies
3. accommodation available in community hospitals

Reasons for delay include: no alternative to acute care; uncoordinated planning; delay in performing needs assessment; not enough beds in community hospitals and funding or workforce shortfalls. Recommendations to the Department of Health include:

- robust data collection
- increase recruitment of occupational therapists and physiotherapists
- take a proactive stance in noting common difficulties and advising health and social care communities how these may be overcome.

Recommendations to NHS trusts include:

- make discharge policy widely known
- plan as early as possible and map 'patient journeys' to avoid bottlenecks
- involve patients and carers in planning
- monitor emergency readmissions
- PCTs to monitor organisation of equipment services
- increase use of independent sector providers

Strategic Health Authorities to maintain a clear picture of what services are available and communicate this widely.

National Audit Office (2003) *Developing effective services for older people: report by the Comptroller and Auditor General: HC518: session 2002-3.* London: The Stationery Office

Summary: directed at Government departments, this report looks at all public services including: health and social care, transport, housing, information, leisure, education, pensions and benefits. It focuses on five specific initiatives: the *Inter-ministerial Group for Older People* now the *Cabinet Committee on Older People;* a government-wide programme called *Better government for older people*; a report *Winning the generation game (2002)*; the *NSF for older people (2001)* and a strategic framework *Quality and choice for older people's housing (2000)* based on a series of 'listening events'. In view of the ageing of UK population, the report estimates the cost of pensions and services at 8% of the GDP. Recommendations include:

- a plan for an *Older People Strategy* urging coordination between the Cabinet Committee on Older People and the Department of Work and Pensions
- Cabinet Committee should repeat their 'listening exercise' and report more publicly their findings as without feedback there can be disillusionment
- all Departments to consider appointing champions and for them to work with the Department of Work and Pensions to coordinate all work concerning older people's issues
- Department of Health to make clear who the champions of older people are within the NHS, thus providing stronger leadership
- better coordination needed between the Departments and HM Treasury and closer working between Departments of Health and Work and Pensions
- Departments of Health and Work and Pensions well placed to commission and coordinate research. Recommends involving National Collaboration on Ageing Research and Funders' Forum for Research on Ageing and Older People

Further reading:

Cabinet Office Performance and Innovation Unit (2000) *Winning the generation game: improving opportunities for people aged 50-65 in work and community activity.* London: The Stationery Office

Department of Environment, Transport and the Regions and Department of Health (2001) *Quality and choice for older people's housing: a strategic framework.* London: DETR

Older People's Commissioners Bill. (2004) London: The Stationery Office

Summary: this would provide for the establishment of commissioners for England and Wales to protect and further the rights of older people. The commissioners would encourage consideration of older people's interests, advise government and investigate complaints or any other matters of interest taking into consideration: health, protection from abuse/neglect, older peoples' contribution to society and social/economic well-being.

National Audit Office (2004) *Welfare to work: tackling the barriers to the employment of older people: report by the Comptroller and Auditor General: HC1206 session 2003-04.* London: The Stationery Office

Summary: there are fewer over-50s working than any other age group and although the UK compares well, this problem is common in Europe as well. Many would like to work but are inhibited from doing so because of ageism, lack of relevant skills or experience, lack of confidence, health problems or the conditions of the local labour market. The report discusses the benefits all round of being in work; the Government's Welfare to Work strategy that includes employment programmes, flexible retirement, training schemes and moves to tackle ageism and promote diversity. These schemes affect and involve every Government department. The report makes recommendations for future progression to Jobcentre Plus, the Learning and Skills Council, Departments of Works and Pensions and of Trade and Industry and to the Cabinet Committee on Older People to ensure coordination.

House of Commons Health Committee (2004) *Elder abuse: second report of session 2003-4: HC111-I.* London: The Stationery Office

Summary: elder abuse is an under-reported, hidden problem that can involve financial, drug, sexual and physical abuse as well as neglect. The report's first concern is to determine the extent of the problem and establish a clear definition that can be applied and used by all state and charitable institutions. Further recommendations include:

- increase inspection visits to NHS care homes
- for concerns with over-medication: draw attention to the *NSF (2001)* recommendation that drug regimes are reviewed at least yearly and every six months for multiple drug users
- vulnerable adult protection committees set up within every local authority
- these committees to address the issue of financial abuse in their policies; the report also supports the proposed *Mental Capacity Bill (2004)* in its provision to prevent people abusing power of attorney
- CHAI and CSCI to work together to regulate and protect the health needs of older adults in social care provision
- certification of a death in a care home should be done by independent GP, not a GP-owner/manager of the home; GP retainer fees should be abolished

Further reading:
Chatterjee, M. (2003) Inquiry turns spotlight on elder abuse. *Nursing Times* 99(49)10-11

Nolan, M. (2004) Elder abuse: a wake-up call to nurse educationalists. *British Journal of Nursing* 13(9) 510

Philp, I. (2004) *Better health in old age.* London: Department of Health

Summary: a progress report looking at the impact on older people's health of the *NSF for older people (2001)*. Notes increasing uptake of 'flu jabs' and breast screening, reduction in delayed discharges, improved convalescent care, and an increase in stroke units in England. Other sections focus on

- person-centred care improving with direct payments and greater choice
- joined-up services: a single assessment process and integrated care for falls, stroke, mental health and incontinence; mental health still a major issue although suicides have dropped
- timely response to needs: future services will be looking to be proactive with screening, 'anticipatory care' and early intervention, helping to avoid crises later
- new developments: looking at the use of telecare and the work of the 1,800 older people's champions in trusts and councils

Audit Commission (2004) *Older people: independence and well-being: the challenge for public services.* London: Audit Commission

Summary: looks at the changes public services will have to make with regard to the independence and welfare of older people. Considers the issues that are of most concern to older people including:

- a safe comfortable home
- good neighbourhoods, close to friends and amenities
- social interaction and networking
- getting about
- income and 'paying their way'
- access to good information and
- keeping healthy

These refer to the majority of older people who don't need care services as well as the minority of frail older people who do. The report is divided into five chapters, each a separate report as follows:

1. older people's views about what they need to live independent lives
2. examples of good strategic practice from some local authorities
3. how a focus on independence can improve the lives of the frail and disabled by taking a proactive approach and using new technologies
4. the vital role of carers
5. an agenda for success

Recommendations to councils include:

- planning beyond care services to address older people's priorities as expressed above
- involving and empowering older people
- keeping informed about their local population and future trends
- offering a range of services including proactive support
- tackling ageism
- supporting carers

Supplementary Reading

Bainbridge, I. and Ricketts, A. (2003) *Improving older people's services: an overview of performance.* London: Social Services Inspectorate, Department of Health

Bowers, Helen et al (1999) *Standards for health and social care standards for older people.* London: Health Advisory Service 2000 and Brighton: Pavilion Publishing

British Geriatrics Society (2003) *Standards of medical care for older people: expectations and recommendations.* London: BGS

Cornwell, Jocelyn (1989) *The consumer's view: elderly people and community health services.* London: King's Fund

Crampton, J. and Ricketts, S. (2002) *A catalyst for change: driving change in the strategic commissioning of non-acute services for older people.* London: Department of Health

Department of Health (2001) *Care homes for older people: national minimum standards and the care home regulations.* London: The Stationery Office

Department of Health (2000) *Out in the open: breaking down the barriers for older people.* London: Department of Health

DHSS Inspectorate (1995) *The abuse of older people in domestic settings.* London: HMSO

Easterbrook, Lorna (1999) *When we are very old: reflections on treatment, care and support of older people.* London: King's Fund

Edwards, Margaret (2000) *Primary care groups and older people: signs of progress.* London: King's Fund

Finch, Jenny and Orrell, Martin (1999) *Standards for mental health services for older people.* London: Health Advisory Service 2000 and Brighton: Pavilion Publishing

Fruin, David for the Social Services Inspectorate (2000) *Getting the right break: inspection of short-term breaks for people with physical disabilities and older people.* London: Department of Health

Glendinning, C. Davies, B. Pickard, L. and Comas-Herrera, A. (2004) *Funding long-term care for older people: lessons from other countries.* London: Joseph Rowntree Foundation

Glendinning, C, (2004) *Support for carers of older people: some intranational and national comparisons: a review of the literature prepared for the Audit Commission.* London: Audit Commission

Hornstein, Zmira et al (2001) *Outlawing age discrimination: foreign lessons, UK choices.* Bristol: The Policy Press for the Joseph Rowntree Foundation

Levenson, R. (2003) *Auditing age discrimination: a practical approach to promoting age equality in health and social care.* London: King's Fund

Margiotta, P. et al (2003) *Are you listening: Current practice in information, advice and advocacy services for older people.* York: Joseph Rowntree Foundation

Qureshi, H. et al (1998) *Overview: outcomes of social care for older people and carers.* London: Social Policy Research Unit

Roberts, Emilie (2000) *Improving services for older people: what are the issues for primary care groups?* London: King's Fund

Robinson, Janice (2002) *Age equality in health and social care.* London: Institute for Public Policy Research and the Nuffield Foundation

Royal College of Nursing (1998) *What a difference a nurse makes: an RCN report on the benefits of expert nursing to the clinical outcomes in the continuing care of older people.* London: Royal College of Nursing

Royal College of Nursing (1999) *Restraint revisited: rights, risks and responsibility: guidance for nurses working with older people.* London: RCN

Social Services Inspectorate and Department of Health (1995) *Moving on: report of the national inspection of social services department arrangements for the discharge of older people from hospital to residential or nursing home care.* London: Department of Health

UKCC (1997) *The nursing and health visiting contribution to the continuing care of older people.* London: UKCC

Wade, Barbara (1996) *The changing face of community care for older people: whose choice?* London: Royal College of Nursing

Walker, Alan (1994) *Half a century of promises: the failure to realise community care for older people.* London: Counsel and Care

Wittenberg, R. Comas-Herrera, A. Pickard, L. and Hancock, R. (2004) *Future demand for long-term care in the UK: a summary of projections of long-term finance for older people to 2051.* London: Joseph Rowntree Foundation

6 Midwifery

House of Commons Health Committee (1992) *Second report: maternity services, volume 1.* (chair Nicholas Winterton) London: HMSO

Summary: the main outcome of this report is the shift towards 'woman-centred' care and the establishment of the Expert Maternity Group responsible for the subsequent report *Changing childbirth (1993)*. The first chapters trace the history of maternity services this century and consider evidence from organisations (such as the National Childbirth Trust), health professionals and mothers. Previously, women were urged to give birth in hospital maternity units in the mistaken belief that this was safer. The report refutes this belief, advising against the assumption that this is what women want and advocating instead the 'three Cs':

- CONTINUITY: of place of antenatal care and birth with known individual midwife
- CHOICE: sufficient information given to enable woman to determine where to give birth and what care she wants (feeding methods, epidurals, caesareans etc)
- CONTROL: women to be able to talk with health professionals and contribute to the decisions about their care during all stages of pregnancy and birth

The report stresses that women's rights take precedence over those of health professionals who must do more to implement the three Cs.

Community-based care to be encouraged: antenatal visits to be made in the home and the systematic closure of rural maternity units to stop.

Maternity care is set in the broad socio-economic context taking into account factors such as diet and maternity leave and considering financial implications such as of providing benefits and income support during pregnancy.

The implications for training are considered (of GPs, obstetricians and midwives), as well as research (National Perinatal Epidemiology Unit) and statistics (of neonatal morbidity and birthweight).

The report recommends that the expertise and status of midwives be recognised, team midwifery be established and midwives given the right to admit women to hospital.

Further reading:

Garrod, D. (1994) Cutting the cord. *Modern Midwife* 4(2) 31-3

Meldrum, P. (1994) Moving towards a common understanding in maternity services. *Midwifery* 10(4) 165-70

Rothwell, R. (1996) Changing childbirth. *Midwives* 109(1306) 291-4

Walton, I. (1994) Adapt and evolve. *Nursing Times* 90(32) 56-7

Department of Health (1993) *Changing childbirth: Part 1: report of the expert maternity group.* (chair Julia Cumberlege) *Part II: Survey of good communications practice in maternity services.* London: HMSO

Summary: an Expert Maternity Group was set up in response to the House of Commons Health Select Committee report *Maternity services (1992)* to review policy on NHS maternity care, particularly during childbirth, and to make recommendations. The objective of the group was to improve NHS maternity services. Report identifies three key principles which must underlie effective woman-centred maternity services and gives the objectives and action points to be met by the purchasers and providers of maternity services. The key principles are:

- the woman is the focus of maternity care. She should be able to feel that she is in control of what is happening to her and able to make decisions about her care, based on her needs, having discussed them fully with the professionals involved

- maternity services must be readily and easily accessible to all. They should be sensitive to the needs of the local population and based primarily in the community

- women should be involved in the monitoring and planning of maternity services to ensure that they are responsive to the needs of a changing society. In addition care should be effective and resources used efficiently

The theme of the report is: 'woman-centred care, control, choice and continuity' with an emphasis on the role the midwife is to play in maternity care.

Further reading:
Everitt, N. (1995) Implementing good practice: the Changing Childbirth implementation team. *British Journal of Midwifery* 3(3) 139-41

Jackson, K. (1995) Changing childbirth: encouraging debate. *British Journal of Midwifery* 3(3) 137-8

Locock, L. and Dopson, S. (2001) when push comes to shove. *Health Service Journal* 111(5737) 28-9

Savage, W. (1994) The Mabel Liddiard Memorial Lecture, 1994. Changing childbirth: would Mabel Liddiard approve? *Midwives Chronicle* 107(1282) 411-3

Department of Health (1994) *The patient's charter: maternity services.* London: HMSO

Summary: outlines patients' rights in relation to maternity services, concentrating specifically on: midwifery, obstetrics and paediatrics services; maternity records; antenatal appointments; security in maternity units; pregnancy care.
The document also gives a very brief outline of some of the improvements in maternity services implemented since the publication of *Changing childbirth (1993)*.

Audit Commission (1997) *First class delivery: improving maternity services in England and Wales.* London: Audit Commission

Summary: this report is the result of surveys carried out amongst maternity care professionals and recent mothers and is aimed mostly at purchasers of maternity care. It looks at how 'woman-centred care' services recommended in *Changing Childbirth*

(1993) have been implemented and takes into consideration the impact of clinical effectiveness information and regional differences in services. There are chapters on antenatal, perinatal and postnatal services from the woman's perspective and also from the point of view of service providers. Each chapter ends with recommendations for improvement for trusts, commissioners of services and the NHS Executive.

The central themes are:

- effectiveness information for clinicians and midwives
- improved choice and information for women
- continuity of care and increased role for midwives
- following best practice

Further reading:
Fitzsimmons B (1997) First class delivery: a review of the Audit Commission report. *British Journal of Midwifery* 5(7) 388-92

Robinson J (1997) First class delivery: auditing the auditors. *British Journal of Midwifery* 5(4) 227

Department of Health (1998) *Midwifery: delivering our future: report by the Standing Nursing and Midwifery Advisory Committee.* (chair Alison Norman) London: Department of Health.

Summary: the theme of the report is the evolving role of the midwifery profession. Changes in maternity services during the 1990s are outlined and their impact on education, supervision, autonomy and professional role of midwives. Influencing factors include woman-centred care, primary care-led NHS, midwives' role in management and cooperation with obstetricians and GPs.

Recommendations include:

- midwifery education should be at graduate level while maintaining shortened courses for registered nurses
- representation of midwives on education purchasing consortia
- access for midwives to clinical effectiveness information
- midwife involvement in management of trusts and commissioners to encourage woman-centred care
- NHS research and development organisations to encourage research in midwifery
- opportunities for professional development and lifelong learning to be available to all midwives
- consideration should be given to prescribing by midwives

Further reading:
Henderson, C. (1998) Midwifery: delivering our future. *British Journal of Midwifery* 6(5) 292-3

Association of Radical Midwives (1999) *Vision for midwifery education.* London: ARM

Summary: a vision influenced by factors such as: direct entry training; the move to higher education institutions; students' supernumerary status; practising midwives ill-prepared for new kind of students; tutors isolated from clinical practice; attrition rates of between 5 and 15%. In ARM's view:

- midwifery education should aim to develop midwives who are able to attend any woman in any social context and regardless of class, sexuality or creed
- the profession should be looking to attract women with a sense of vocation
- "visionary midwifery" depends on non-hierarchical relationships and this should form the basis of midwifery education

ARM stresses the importance of pregnant women valuing themselves as birthing women and of babies coming into the world in optimal emotional circumstances. It follows that students must learn to develop strong 'personal, interpersonal, psychomotor, critical and analytical skills' as well as learning to be health care providers in the context of maternity care. Their model for teaching and learning should be based on a 'caseload and apprenticeship' style involving:

- one-to-one and group learning
- enquiry-based learning
- role play
- shared learning
- information technology

Assessment should be via case studies, exams, oral presentation and three-way (midwife, tutor, student) practical assessment. The report ends by outlining the roles of mentors and lecturer-practitioners.

Royal College of Midwives (2000) *Vision 2000.* London: Royal College of Midwives

Summary: the 'vision' concerns the development of UK maternity services in the light of the new health policies. Whilst models of care vary across the country, the RCM proposes twelve key principles to inform future development. These include:

- woman and family-centred care
- public health: reducing morbidity and promoting equality of access
- community focused care 'seamlessly' integrated with acute services
- pregnancy and birth to be viewed as a normal state of health, avoiding unnecessary medicalisation
- midwifery-led care: whilst working in partnership with other professionals and care agencies, strong midwifery leadership will ensure high quality and continuity of care

Further reading:
Gould, D. (2000) Stronger leadership is needed before we can 'own' change. *British Journal of Midwifery* 8(8) 480-81

Ball, L. Curtis, P. and Kirkham, M. (2002) *Why do midwives leave?* London: Royal College of Midwives

Summary: instigated by the national shortage of midwives, a research study that looked at why midwives leave the profession and what might encourage them to return. Findings:

- the decision to leave was painful and not made 'in a hurry'
- 30% of respondents gave 'dissatisfaction with midwifery' as their reason for leaving. Other reasons include: family commitments, retirement, ill health. career change. For these other groups, dissatisfaction with midwifery was also a major issue.
- younger and newly qualified midwives felt a conflict between what they had studied for and actual practice
- rotation in clinical areas leaves midwives feeling 'dislocated', undermining their confidence and making it hard to hold and sustain relationships with colleagues and clients
- midwives felt unsupported by management and worse, reported intimidation
- workplace stress is widespread and whilst midwives found colleagues supportive, these relationships were easily undermined

What would induce midwives to return to practice?

- effective, resourced support that values their skills and experience
- flexible working for those with families
- debate needed about the necessity to rotate around all clinical areas
- whilst pay was not as big an issue as expected, improved prospects for promotion and professional development would encourage midwives

The report ends with recommendations covering: patterns of working; managerial support; culture of midwifery; education-practice gap; recruitment and retention; pay and promotion and the impact all of this has on mothers.

Further reading:
Rosser, J. (2001) Serving two masters. *Health Care Risk Report* 7(6) 18-9

House of Commons Health Committee (2003) *Provision of maternity services: fourth report of session 02-03: HC464-1.* London: The Stationery Office

Summary: looks at provision of services in England, in particular focusing on: maternity units, caesarean sections, staffing, and training of those who advise mothers.

Findings include:

- data collection patchy and inconsistent
- women poorly informed and supported about procedure and reasons for caesarean section
- continuity of care is most essential factor in making childbirth a positive experience for women
- inadequate staffing can lead to gaps in the team's skill mix
- maternity staff training essential, less skilled and experienced doctors are more likely to intervene unnecessarily in labour

House of Commons Health Committee (2003) *Choice in maternity services: ninth report of session 02-03 HC796-1.* London The Stationery Office

Summary: based on evidence from an extensive range of professional bodies, experts and pressure groups, the report opens by examining what it means to have 'choice' and looks at a survey conducted at University of Leeds that found that whilst whilst women appeared to have more choice than their predecessors, about 60% of women did not feel in control of what was happening; choice of itself did not necessarily bring a positive outcome - perhaps because of increased obstetric intervention; many women elected for epidurals, because they feared they would not cope without.

Overall conclusions:

- measuring clinical outcome is not always the best measure of success
- a high extent of interventions mitigates against true choice
- when first pregnant, some women find it hard to circumnavigate the 'GP route' to maternity services; not even NHS Direct gives the right advice
- a midwife should be a woman's first port-of-call and:
- a GP's first step should be to make at least one appointment with a community midwife - this to go into the Maternity Standard of the NSF for children, young people and maternity services
- if Department of Health is truly committed to offering choice and de-medicalisation of childbirth then they must work against the closure of the smaller maternity units
- home birth should be promoted
- the NSF is a prime opportunity to recast maternity services away from over medicalisation in acute hospitals, towards choice in a community-led service
- midwifery recruitment a problem, if more home birthing were recommended this may help attract and retain midwives in the profession
- the National Childbirth Trust should specify to pregnant women the minimum tests required - offering prenatal tests doesn't always solve anything and encourages intervention
- women to have the right to choose induction after 41 weeks
- NICE should investigate what would be an appropriate environment for women to deliver their babies
- midwives to have the right to choose not to help with a pool delivery

House of Commons Health Committee (2003) *Inequalities in access to maternity services: eighth report of session 02-03 HC696.* London: The Stationery Office

Summary: good care during pregnancy and immediately after birth is a strong guarantor of good health in later life for mother and child. The report found many individual instances of good practice, some the result of the *Sure Start* programme. Generally however, good practice was not shared or replicated and depended on the initiative of individual mothers. The report looked particularly at women from vulnerable groups such as with mental health problems, disability, homeless etc. In spite of recommendations from *Changing childbirth (1993)* the report found insufficient services for women with severe post-natal depression or affected by disability. Continuity of care was lost through poor communication. Without training and support, staff are ill equipped to help with vulnerable groups; interpreting and BSL services were poor. Recommendations include:

- more research needed, in particular with regard to pregnant women and domestic violence
- interpreters or signers should not be family members
- social workers to discourage women from giving away their babies when there are problems
- midwives should be recruited from different ethnic groups
- pregnant asylum seekers are especially vulnerable and should not be detained for longer than absolutely necessary
- improve support to promote breastfeeding and stopping smoking

Further reading:

Bewley, S. Friend, J. and Mezey, G. (eds) (1997) *Violence against women.* London: Royal College of Obstetrics and Gynaecology

Department of Health (2000) *Domestic violence: a resource manual for health care professionals.* London: Department of Health

Independent Midwives Association (2003) *A solution to the problem: IMA's submission to the Choice, Responsiveness and Equity Group.* London: IMA

Summary: the NHS funds 99% of midwifery care. Despite 'superhuman efforts' that care is flawed because it is determined not by a woman's needs but by what "enables the institute to function". Independent midwifery offers:

- unhurried antenatal care
- labour care with a midwife who has developed a relationship of trust over nine months
- care and support for a month after birth

From 340 births delivered by independent midwives in year 2002-3 there were fewer inductions, caesarean sections, episiotomies and instrumental deliveries compared with births delivered within the NHS for the equivalent period. Whilst recognising such an optimum level of care has to be paid for, the IMA proposes a *NHS Community Midwifery Model* that would enable the NHS to provide this. The model begins with the woman choosing her midwife. The midwife may be employed within a trust or she may be self-employed in which case:

- there would be a national midwifery contract, paying a set fee per woman much as opticians, pharmacists and GPs are contracted for their services in the UK
- standards of care regulated by *NMC Midwives rules and standards (2004)* and practice subject to regular peer review
- contract would include access to all NHS facilities

The submission goes on to cover services for women with special needs such as disability, drug and alcohol problems etc and then outlines the funding arrangements in detail.

Recruitment and retention are examined as there is a national shortage of midwives and many leave the profession. The IMA points to the success this model has had in New Zealand and stresses the benefits including: meeting targets to reduce caesarean sections, increase breastfeeding and thus improve pubic health and reduce incidents of post-natal depression.

MIDIRS (2003/4) *Informed choice.* http://www.infochoice.org/

Summary: based on the best available evidence, *Informed choice* comprises 15 booklets on every aspect of pregnancy and childbirth written for both professionals and clients. This is to promote woman-centred care based on informed and shared decision-making. Topics include: screening, ultrasound scans, waterbirth, diet, pain relief in labour, breast feeding etc.

Department of Education & Skills and Department of Health (2004) *Maternity standard: national service framework for children, young people and maternity services.* London: Department of Health

Summary: part three, standard 11 of the national service framework (NSF) is concerned with providing woman-centred care from pre-conception to three months after birth based on the following 'vision':

Maternity services should be flexible, woman and child-centred, paying particular attention to vulnerable and disadvantaged groups. Support should be for as normal a pregnancy and birth as possible, with medical intervention only if clinically necessary. Midwifery and obstetric care based on providing good clinical and psychological outcomes for mother and baby. The standard continues as follows:

owomen to have access to information and support in order to share the decision-making in her care, including allowing for disclosure and support in cases of domestic violence

- care pathways to integrate maternity and neonatal services
- optimum health for the woman and her partners to be seen as key to preconception care. Women to have direct access to midwife and screening
- care should address mental health issues during and after pregnancy
- women to choose the place for her delivery with facilities to transfer in case of complications; caesarean section to be offered on basis of clinical need only
- whoever present at a birth to be skilled in neonatal resuscitation
- well-planned post-natal care to be provided following a structured assessment
- women to be supported in breast feeding
  The standard notes seven markers of good practice:
- facilitate normal delivery where possible
- women to be involved in planning her own care and in the broader context in planning and reviewing all local maternity services
- service to be proactive in engaging women, especially from minority and disadvantaged groups

- there should be integrated, 'networked' maternity and neonatal services
- maternity services to be networked to include the care of women with complex needs and women with their partners who smoke or are substance mis-users
- service to promote breastfeeding but to support women whatever their choice

Further reading:
Cresswell, J. (2002) How should the NSF improve maternity services? *Health Care Risk Report* 8(3) 14-5

Nursing and Midwifery Council (2004) *Midwives rules and standards.* London: NMC

Summary: these have a statutory basis in the *Nursing and Midwifery Council (Midwives) Rules Order of Council 2004* and come into force on August 2004. They describe what can be expected from professional, registered midwives and their supervisors and are arranged as follows:

- midwives giving notice of intention to practice to supervising authorities
- authorities publishing details of practising midwives and forwarding them to the NMC register
- suspensions from practice where there are concerns about a midwife's competence
- responsibility and sphere of practice: outlines the limits of a midwife's responsibilities and at what point she must refer in emergencies
- administration of medicines
- protocols for participating in clinical trials
- record-keeping
- inspections of practice, equipment and premises
- becoming a midwifery supervisor
- scope of practice for named supervisors
- the roles of the local supervising authority (LSA) midwifery officers
- LSA to publish details of their procedures and annual report

Further reading:
The Nursing and Midwifery Council (Midwives) Rules Order of Council 2004: statutory instrument 2004 no. 1746. London: The Stationery Office

Supplementary Reading

Abortion Act 1967: chapter 87. London: HMSO

Chamberlain, G. (ed) (1994) *The future of maternity services.* London: Royal College of Obstetricians and Gynaecologists.

Congenital Disabilities (Civil Liability) Act 1976: chapter 28. London: HMSO

Department of Health. *Confidential enquiry into stillbirths and deaths in infancy (annual).* London: The Stationery Office

Department of Health. *Report on confidential enquiries into maternal deaths in the UK (triennial).* London: The Stationery Office

Department of Health (1997) *Learning together: professional education for maternity care*. London: The Stationery Office

Department of Health (1998) *Why mothers die: report on confidential enquiries into maternal deaths in the UK 1994-1996*. London The Stationery Office

English National Board (1998) *Creating lifelong learners: partnerships for care: guidelines for pre-registration midwifery programmes of education*. London: ENB

Garcia, J. (1993) *Getting consumers' views of maternity care: examples of how the OPCS survey manual can help*. London: HMSO

Human Fertilisation and Embryology Act 1990: chapter 37. London: HMSO

Maternity Alliance (1999) *Maternity services for women with learning difficulties: a report of a partnership of midwives, community nurses and parents*. London: Maternity Alliance

Maternity Care Working Party (2001) *Modernising maternity care: a commissioning toolkit for primary care trusts in England*. London: RCOG

Redshaw, M. (1996) *Delivering neonatal care: the neonatal unit as a working environment: a survey of neonatal unit nursing*. London: HMSO

Royal College of Midwives (2002) *Midwives: the backbone of UK maternity services. London: RCM*

Royal College of Obstetrics and Gynaecology (2001) *The care of women requesting abortion*. London: RCOG

Royal College of Obstetrics and Gynaecology and Royal College of Midwives (1999) *Towards safer childbirth: minimum standards for the organisation of labour wards: report of a joint working party*. London: RCOG

Royal College of Obstetrics and Gynaecology (2001) *Why mothers die: report on confidential enquiries into maternal deaths in the UK 1997-2000*. London: RCOG

Still-Birth (Definition) Act 1992: chapter 29. London: HMSO

7 **Children and Young People**

Children Act 1989: chapter 41 London: HMSO

Summary: a comprehensive piece of legislation that seeks to protect the welfare of children by striking a balance between children's rights, parental responsibilities and the duty of the state to protect children who are at risk. The roles of welfare agencies and their relationships with parents are defined. Areas such as: day care, adoption, protection orders, children's homes, fostering and so on are legislated for. The Act came into force in 1991.

Further reading:
Gaskins, Richard (1993) Comprehensive reform in child welfare: the British Children Act 1989 *Social Service Review* 67(1) 1-15

Kent, Paul et al (1990) Guide to the Children Act 1989. *Community Care* 19.4.1990 supplement

Rickford, Frances (1992) Happy families. *Social Work Today* 23(38) 20

Department of Health and Royal College of Nursing (1992) *The Children Act 1989: what every nurse, health visitor and midwife needs to know.* London: HMSO

Hogg, Christine (1989) *The NAWCH quality review: setting standards for children in health care.* London: National Association for the Welfare of Children in Hospital

Summary: a document offering principles and checklists for setting standards on all aspects of child health care including: in-patients, outpatients, accident and emergency departments, diagnostic and support services and preventive child health. Examples of consumer surveys are given. The review notes three principles behind promoting good hospital and health care for children:

- the involvement of parents
- conducive surroundings/ward environment
- good communication between staff and children and their parents

and gives the NAWCH 'Charter' as a basis for standard setting. The Charter makes ten statements about the care of children in hospital, most of which have subsequently made their way into the *Patient's charter: services for children and young people (1996).* They include that children should be hospitalised only when necessary; they have the right to have their parents with them as much as possible; they are entitled to information and to be involved in decisions about their treatment; the services should be geared to their needs and they should be treated by specially trained staff.

Further reading:
Galvin, June and Leonard A. Goldstone (1988) *Junior monitor: an index of the quality of nursing care for junior citizens on hospital wards.* Newcastle upon Tyne: Newcastle upon Tyne Polytechnic Products Ltd

Siddle, J. (1991) A voice for children...NAWCH the National Association for the Welfare of Children in Hospital. *British Journal of Theatre Nursing* 1(6) 4-5

NAWCH (1990) *Setting standards for adolescents in hospital.* London: National Association for the Welfare of Children in Hospital

Summary: the report starts with the recognition that adolescents have needs separate from children and adults, the word implying change in every sense and a growing need for individuality, autonomy and independence. Purchasers and providers are invited to give consideration to: specialised staffing, the need for privacy, links with the outside, a flexible day and so on. The report gives examples of good practice and a "charter for care".

Further reading:
Shelley, H. (1993) Adolescent needs in hospital. *Paediatric Nursing* 5(9) 16-8

Department of Health (1991) *Welfare of children and young people in hospital.* London: HMSO

Summary: this report identifies issues which providers of health services to children need to address in the light of the new structure of purchasers and providers implemented after Working for patients (1989). It contains recommendations for good practice and areas covered include the unique needs of children in hospital, staff and training needs, day and community services, consent to treatment and parental involvement.

Further reading:
Rogers, Rosemary (1991) Action for sick children. *Paediatric Nursing* 3(90) 6-7
Shelley, Pauline (1991) A commitment to children. *Paediatric Nursing* 3(7) 10-11

Thornes, R (1991) *Just for the day: children admitted to hospital for day treatment.* London: Caring for Children in the Health Services.

Summary: this document looks specifically at day case treatment in the overall context of children's health services. It makes recommendations for both purchasers and providers and outlines twelve recommended quality standards in areas such as: admission procedures, environment, nursing support after discharge and parental responsibilities.

Further reading:
Norris, C. (1992) Making the day bearable. *Paediatric Nursing* 4(3) 21-2
Thornes, Rosemary (1992) A spur to action. *Paediatric Nursing* 4(5) 6-7
While, Alison and Janet Crawford (1992) Day surgery: expediency or quality care? *Paediatric Nursing* 4(3) 18-20

Department of Health (1992) *Child protection: guidance for senior nurses, health visitors and midwives.* London: HMSO

Summary: this report outlines where responsibilities lie for child protection by health authorities, senior nurses and other health care staff. It was written in the context of recent legislation such as the *Children Act 1989* and the *NHS and Community Care Act*

1990. It looks at issues surrounding child abuse and protection in general, and in specific settings such as accident and emergency, school nursing, learning disabilities. Contains examples of good practice.

Department of Health (1993) *The rights of the child: a guide to the UN convention.* London: Department of Health

Summary: sets out the rights of children and young people as laid down by the United Nations convention on the rights of the child to which the UK agreed to be bound in 1991. The Government declares its support for the Convention with certain reservations. There is guidance for the public about who to approach if they feel the rights of children are not being met. Units have been set up to monitor adherence to the Convention; their addresses are listed.

Further reading:

Fulton, Yvonne (1996) Children's rights and the role of the nurse. *Paediatric Nursing* 8(10) 29-31

General Assembly of the United Nations (1989) *Convention on the rights of the child.* New York: United Nations

Newell, P. (1993) *The UN convention and children's rights in the UK.. 2nd ed* London: National Children's Bureau.

Audit Commission (1993) *Children first: a study of hospital services.* London: HMSO

Summary: although child care in hospital has been discussed and legislated for since 1959, the report states, the service can still fail and its effectiveness is often not questioned. Six principles are identified:

- child and family-centred care
- specially skilled staff
- separate facilities
- effective treatment
- appropriate hospitalisation
- strategic commissioning

Further reading:
Bailey, J. (1996) Children first: the local audit. *Paediatric Nursing* 8(3) 6-7

Thornes, Rosemary (1993) *Bridging the gaps: an exploratory study of the interfaces between primary and specialist care for children within the health service.* London: Caring for Children in the Health Services

Summary: a research study that looks at the quality of care provision as the child moves from one agency to another within the health service. It directs its statements and recommendations at GPs, commissioners and providers of care, the NHS Management Executive and the Department of Health and these include a need for:

- shared information and knowledge
- equity of service

- the service to be delivered as close as possible to home
- parents to be clear about who is providing what service and what care they themselves must provide

Further reading:
Rogers, Rosemary (1993) A seamless service? *Paediatric Nursing* 5(2) 5

Hogg, Christine (1994) *Setting standards for children undergoing surgery.* London: Action for Sick Children

Summary: the report offers thirteen standards to purchasers and providers of child care in surgery. These include: the need for specially skilled staff, consent to treatment, preparation for the operation, parents visiting the anaesthetic and recovery rooms, post-operative care, and discharge procedures.

Department of Health (1994) *The health of the nation: a handbook on child and adolescent mental health.* London: HMSO

Summary: this booklet states that while severe mental illness is rare in children and adolescents, between 10 and 20% may need help with mental health problems. Untreated problems cause distress to the child and all who care for them and can lead to severe problems in adulthood as well as an increased demand on public services. The guide offers an action plan for providers, a prevalence table of problems (anorexia, enuresis, phobias etc) and a list of contacts.

Further reading:
Whitfield, W. (1995) Stemming the rising tide. *Paediatric Nursing* 7(4) 16-7

The Allitt inquiry: independent inquiry relating to the deaths and injuries on the children's ward at Grantham and Kesteven General Hospital during the period February to April 1991. (1994) (chair C. Clothier) London: HMSO

Summary: the document details the circumstances leading up to the killing of four children and injury to nine children by nurse Beverley Allitt in the spring of 1991. Each incident is documented together with the responses to the attacks. Beverley Allitt's training into the profession and her subsequent appointment to the children's ward are discussed as well as staffing levels and ward management at the time of the incidents. In the light of the findings, thirteen recommendations are made including several in the area of nurse recruitment.

Further reading:
Leenders, F. (1995) Malevolent intervention. *Paediatric Nursing* 7(9) 6-7

Lunn, J. (1994) Implications of the Allitt inquiry...pre-employment health screening and its relationship to psychiatric illness. *British Journal of Nursing* 3(5) 201-2

MacDonald, A. (1995) Lest we forget. *Paediatric Nursing* 7(9) 10-11

MacDonald, A. (1996) Responding to the results of the Beverley Allitt inquiry. *Nursing Times* 92(2) 23-5

Rogers, R. (1994) Lessons to be learned...on the inquiry team into the Allitt Tragedy. *Nursing Standard* 8(29) 18-9

Royal College of Nursing (1994) *The care of sick children: a review of the guidelines in the wake of the Allitt inquiry.* London: Royal College of Nursing

Audit Commission (1994) *Seen but not heard: co-ordinating community child health and social services for children in need: detailed evidence and guidelines for managers and practitioners.* London: HMSO

Summary: this report reviews the problems that have arisen between health and social services in the provision of child care as a result of the NHS and Community Care Act 1990. A plan of action is proposed to ensure a closer collaboration and includes the introduction of joint child service plans. The report focuses on the areas of child protection, children looked after by social services, immunisation, family support, day care and child health surveillance.

Further reading:
Notter, J. (1994) Audit Commission report leaves many questions unanswered. *British Journal of Nursing* 3(12) 596-7

Professional Briefing 3 (1995) Co-ordinating community child health services. *Health Visitor* 68(3) 112-5

Department of Health (1996) *The patient's charter: services for children and young people.* London: Department of Health

Summary: a booklet outlining the rights, standards and expectations of children in health and sickness and with special needs. They include the right to see a doctor in confidence; the right to explanations and involvement in discussions and decisions about treatment, the right to be accompanied by a parent when in hospital, and to a named nurse, education, effective pain relief, nice food and so on.

Further reading:
Glasper E.A. and Powell, C. (1996) The challenge of the children's charter: rhetoric vs reality. *British Journal of Nursing* 5(1) 26-9

Leenders, F. (1996) An overview of policies guiding health care for children. *Nursing Standard* 10(28) 33-8

Moores, Y. (1996) What's new for children?...the new patient's charter and services for children. *Nursing Standard* 10(26) 20-1

Hogg, Christine (1996) *Health services for children and young people: a guide for commissioners and providers.* London: Action for Sick Children

Summary: this pack of four booklets update the NAWCH: *Setting standards for children in health care (1989).*They cover: principles for commissioning and providing services; health promotion, illness and disability and examples of audit with checklists. Good practice is promoted in key areas such as hospital services, child health services in the community and child and adolescent mental health. The document emphasises the importance of recognising children's specific needs and of cooperation between health authorities and social services.

Further reading:
Rogers, R. (1996) Health authorities fail to get the message...new guidance on commissioning health services for children and young people. *Paediatric Nursing* 8(1) 3

Hogg, Christine (1997) *Emergency services for children and young people: a guide for commissioners and providers.* London: Action for Sick Children

Summary: although children and young people are major users of emergency services, few hospitals make special arrangements by providing suitably qualified staff or a child friendly environment. The report proposes an unbroken chain of care covering primary care, accident and emergency departments, children's services and child and adolescent mental health services. There should be a trained children's nurse available in the accident and emergency department for all shifts and suitably qualified and experienced medical staff available at all times. A dedicated mental health team should be on call. Practical advice is given for commissioners on principles of emergency services, community emergencies, accident and emergency departments and ambulance services. There are audit checklists and questionnaires designed to obtain feedback from patients and their families.

Further reading:
New guidance on emergency services. (1997) *Paediatric Nursing* 9(6) 4

Scott, G. (1997) Children in need. *Nursing Standard* 11(40) 14

Royal College of Paediatrics and Child Health (1997) *Withholding or withdrawing life saving treatment in children.* (chair Neil McIntosh) London: Royal College of Paediatrics and Child Health

Summary: a report offering guidelines to the medical profession about when to consider the withdrawal of treatment. Five circumstances are described:
- when the child is brain dead
- when the child is in a persistent vegetative state
- when treatment would delay death but not relieve suffering
- if survival would leave the child with unreasonable disability
- if child and family feel that further treatment would cause unbearable suffering

The report's basis is that the child's interests come first and that every effort must be made to bring about a consensus between doctors, parents and the child.

House of Commons Health Committee (1997) *The specific health needs of children and young people: second report of the Health Committee: session 1996-97: Vol 1: report together with the proceedings of the Committee.* London: The Stationery Office

Summary: emphasises that children's health needs are significantly different from those of adults' but are not given sufficient priority by policy makers and health service professionals. Changes in attitude, not just policy are required. The Committee found that some major recommendations of the Court report had still not been implemented.

Areas of concern are the still high deaths and injuries from road traffic accidents and accidents generally. Recommends that the Department of Health improves data collection and research on childhood accidents and their prevention. Respiratory and infectious diseases are still a problem with the increase in asthma particularly a cause for concern. Although mortality has decreased, children often live longer with chronic conditions that require further care. Mental health problems may be increasing. There is a lack of data on variations in child health by region and social class but the Department of Health is commissioning further research into this. The Committee supports Brititsh Paediatric Association and Association of the British Pharmaceutical Industry recommendations to stop administration of unlicensed or off-label medicines to children. Recommends that the Department of Health should work with the Department of Education and Employment to assist development of services for autistic children. Effective methods of early screening for eye abnormalities should be evaluated.

Further reading:

Roe, M. (1997) Health services for children. *Paediatric Nursing* 9(3) 6-7

Williams, K. (1997) Call for qualified child nurses. *Nursing Standard* 11(24) 14

House of Commons Health Committee (1997) *Health services for children and young people in the community: home and school: third report of the Health Committee: session 1996-97: report together with the proceedings of the Committee.* London: The Stationery Office

Summary: discusses the work of community children's nursing services (CCNS); health services for children at school; legal liability in respect of untoward accidents; respite care; provision of equipment; fragmentation of existing services for children; inter-agency cooperation; combined and integrated child health services. The report summarises the types of education and training available to nurses in relation to child health. It found that very few nurses are qualified in the care of children and of those that are, 25% do not work with children. Not enough is done to capitalise on the skills of qualified nurses, which indicates the low priority given to children's health. Commends the CCNS but found provision varies and calls for expansion. Recommends the gradual expansion to an integrated CCNS that would have 'responsibility for the whole range of children's nursing including health promotion, health assessment and hands on care' and would include mental health nursing for children. CCNS education should be commissioned on the same basis as health visitors and district nurses. Points out the limitations of the existing school health service. The needs of children with chronic health disorders requiring clinical interventions need urgent attention. Recommends the government establishes a Cabinet Sub-Committee on Children and Young People 'to review, develop and co-ordinate the Government's policy and strategy on issues of special concern to children and young people'.

Further reading:

Casey, A. Young, L. Rote, S. (1997) Integrated nursing services for children. *Paediatric Nursing* 9(5) 8

Whiting, M. (1997) Community children's nursing: a bright future? *Paediatric Nursing* 9(4) 6-7

House of Commons Health Committee (1997) *Child and adolescent mental health services: fourth report of the Health Committee: session 1996-97: report together with the proceedings of the Committee.* London: The Stationery Office

Summary: looks at provision of care in child and adolescent mental health services (CAMHS) and recommends improvements to a service which has been neglected as a priority are within the NHS. Examines range and prevalence of relevant conditions found in younger people and discusses external factors affecting mental health. Looks in particular at suicide, conduct disorder, eating disorders and the difficulties in agreeing on definitions of mental health problems. Evidence of some increase in mental health problems.

Provision of CAMHS is unsatisfactory with failures of liaison and coordination between the agencies involved. Current provision is inadequate both in quality and geographical spread. Recommends that service provision be based on four-tier model and that the Department of Health takes active steps to encourage the adoption of this model across the country to reduce problems of commissioning and inter-agency cooperation. The four-tier model sets out four levels of care:

1. primary care
2. mental health professionals working solo
3. multi-disciplinary teams
4. in-patient units and highly specialised clinics

First tier is seen as vital in identifying and preventing problems at an early stage. NHS Executive should collect information on current provision and distribution of specialist services. Department of Health should remedy poor data gathering and assessment. Cabinet sub-committee on children and young people should include mental health. CAMHS and other children's services should be brought closer together in an integrated and combined children's health service.

Further reading:

Hodges, C. (1997) A model for change. *Mental Health Nursing* 17(3) 28-9

Symington, R. (1997) Mental health services for young people: inadequate and patchy. *Paediatric Nursing* 9(7) 6-7

House of Commons Health Committee (1997) *Hospital services for children and young people: fifth report of the Health Committee: session 1996-97: report together with the proceedings of the committee.* London: The Stationery Office

Summary: looks at the extensive advice and guidance available on standards of care and finds that the implementation of this guidance is patchy. Each purchasing health authority should have a lead commissioner for child health services and the report calls for more effective monitoring of health authority decisions; accident and emergency services should have separate facilities and trained staff for children, but these are not universally available; general surgeons should not operate on small numbers of children and children should not be admitted to adult wards; tertiary services should be organised on a regional level for rarer more complex conditions. The report endorses the principles of *The welfare of children and young people in hospital (1991)* and believes that children should not be in hospital unless absolutely necessary. The needs of children are significantly different from adults and there should be a strong managerial and clinical focus on children's needs across the whole hospital. The child must be the focus and the service must be designed to meet their needs and be needs-led. Recommends improved data collection as the information necessary to plan and provide child-centred cost-effective services is often not available. Many hospitals fail to meet Department of Health standards on trained staff and so the report recommends maintaining an increase in training places for children's nurses for at least five years.

National Co-ordinating Group on Paediatric Intensive Care (1997)
Paediatric intensive care "A framework for the future": National Co-ordinating Group on Paediatric Intensive Care Report to the Chief Executive of the NHS Executive. London: NHS Executive

Summary: the current service has developed in an ad hoc, unplanned way and is provided in a range of different settings many of which are very small units. Specialist retrieval units are limited. There are insufficient trained paediatric intensive care (PIC) clinicians and nurses. The report therefore recommends:

- audits of current service to establish the need for PIC
- organisation of service delivery in four types of hospital: district general, lead centres, major acute hospitals and specialist hospitals
- compliance with standards such as training, competencies and facilities for families. An action plan recommends immediate cessation of extra single isolated beds: children needing intensive care should not be nursed on general children's wards
- there should be a designated lead centre in each area: children should not be cared for in centres which do not meet the report's standards
- there should be a twenty four-hour staffed retrieval service in each geographical area
- protocols on service organisation and management should be developed

Further reading:
Chief Nursing Officer (1997) *A bridge to the future: nursing standards, education and workforce planning in paediatric intensive care: report of the Chief Nursing Officer's taskforce.* London: NHS Executive

Utting, William (1997) *People like us: the report of the review of safeguards for children living away from home.* London: The Stationery Office

Summary: this report arose from the revelations of abuse in children's homes over the preceding twenty years. It studies the residents of children's homes, children in foster care, in boarding schools, penal settings and hospitals in an attempt to formulate a protective strategy. It is especially concerned with the welfare of particularly vulnerable groups of children such as children in care, very young children, children with disabilities, children with behavioural and emotional difficulties and children with parents overseas. The report looks at the hazy area of responsibility: when and whether parents, government or local authorities should be legally responsible for children in different specific situations. Another area is how the criminal justice system protects children from abuse, claiming that it does not always do so effectively or with sensitivity.

A protective strategy is proposed, including the following points:

- to deter abusers: a higher entry threshold for paid and voluntary workers
- overall excellence and vigilance towards abuse in management
- effective disciplinary and criminal procedures to deal with offenders
- effective and improved communication between agencies about known offenders and abusers
- a constant striving for excellence

Further reading:
Stuart, M and Baines, C. (2004) *Progress on safeguards for children living away from home.* London: Joseph Rowntree Foundation

Utting, W. (1998) Sir William Utting highlights the important difficult legal issues which affect children living away from home. *Childright* 143 Jan/Feb 1998 2-4

Willow, C. (1997) CROA supports people like us. *Childright* 142 Dec 1997 18

Viner, Russell and Keane, Mark (1998) *Youth matters: evidence-based best practice for the care of young people in hospital.* London: Action for Sick Children

Summary: provision for physical health care for adolescents is poor, with nurse/physician-led services rather than patient-led and very few dedicated adolescent units. The report offers detailed, evidence-based guidelines on commissioning and providing care, looking at the hospital and ward as environments, inpatient services, staffing and education.

Further reading:
Glasper, A. and Cooper, M. (1999) Hospitals need specialist inpatient adolescent units. *British Journal of Nursing* 8(9) 549

Middleton, Sue Ashworth, Karl and Braithwaite, Ian (1999) *Small fortunes: spending on children, childhood poverty and parental sacrifice.* London: Joseph Rowntree Foundation

Summary: the results of a survey focusing on the lifestyles and living standards of British children. Findings include:

- on average children cost £3000 p.a. most of which comes from their own parents
- food takes the largest proportion of spending with significant amounts going on education and almost no difference between boys and girls; spending increases only slightly with age and yet family credit and foster care allowance calculations are age-related which means that younger children can be seriously disadvantaged
- spending varies according to economic circumstances but not as much as expected; average spending is much higher than income support allowances
- a new 'measure of poverty' is described based on items and activities that the majority of parents see as necessities. Significant numbers of children go without because parents can't afford the cost

- parents themselves are more likely to go without than their children, especially lone parents and those that do not work: they will go without clothing, holidays and sometimes food

Further reading:

Boseley, Sarah (1997) Poor parents who go without to feed their children. *The Guardian* 10.7.1997

Wark, P. and Norton, C. (1997) Family fortunes. *The Sunday Times* 13.7.1997

Department of Health (1999) *Protecting children, supporting parents: a consultation document on the physical punishment of children.* London: The Stationery Office

Summary: a consultation document that seeks to modernise the law relating to the physical punishment of children so as to protect children from harm while maintaining parents' rights of 'reasonable chastisement'. It recognises that 'mild physical rebuke' - smacking - is sometimes appropriate but considers where the line should be drawn with physical punishment. The report recommends adopting the European Court of Human Rights guidelines and offers the following factors for consideration:

- reasons for punishment, persons involved, how soon administered after the event, the vulnerability of the child
- the law could state the some forms of punishment can **never** be deemed reasonable for instance using implements such as canes or belts or any punishment likely to cause head injury (including eyes and ears)
- the law could be changed so that the defence of reasonable chastisement is only available in response to less serious charges i.e. in common assault and not actual or grievous bodily harm
- another option would be to make reasonable chastisement available only to parents and no one else *in loco parentis*

Further reading:

Roberts, M. (2000) Protecting children, supporting parents: government consultation on physical punishment. *Childright* 163 Jan/Feb 2000 3-5

Underdown, A. (2000) *Protecting children, supporting parents: a response by The Children's Society.* London: The Children's Society

Department of Health, Home Office, Department for Education and Employment (1999) *Working together to safeguard children.* London: The Stationery Office

Summary: the main framework for these guidelines comes from the *Children Act 1989* and takes into account the *UN Convention on the rights of the child* (ratified by the UK in 1991) and also the *European Convention on Human Rights.* The guidelines are very detailed and aimed at anyone whose work involves them with children and families i.e. the police, the probation service, education, health and social services etc. They stress that all agencies must work together for the welfare and protection of the child. The guidelines include:

- summaries of lessons learnt from cases of abuse and neglect
- advice about how best to operate the child protection processes such as when concerns about a child are raised, when a child is suffering harm, what to do if a child is away from home, what to do if a tragedy occurs, the principles to be followed when working with children and families
- advice about the roles and responsibilities of all those involved, the importance of effective communication and the need for multi-agency training

Further reading:
Department of Health (2001) *Safeguarding children in whom illness is induced or fabricated by carers with parenting responsibilities: supplementary guidance to Working together to safeguard children.* London: Department of Health

Martin, G. (1998) Working together - a consultation paper too far? *Family Law* September 532-41

Morrison, T. (2000) Working together to safeguard children: challenges and changes for inter-agency coordination. *Journal of Interprofessional Care* 14(4) 363-73

Protection of Children Act 1999: chapter 14. London: The Stationery Office

Summary: this Act requires the Secretary of State for Health to keep a Protection of Children Act List of individuals considered unsuitable to work with children or persons with mental impairment. This used to be a non-statutory 'Consultancy Index List'; the Act makes it statutory but also creates a right of appeal to a new tribunal against inclusion on the list. The Department of Education and Employment has run a similar statutory *List 99* and the two lists will be checked together in a 'one stop' system. The Act amends part 5 of *The Police Act 1977* to allow the Criminal Records Bureau to disclose the criminal records of anyone included on either list. This will make it easier to check on applicants for child care positions.

Further reading:
Corbitt, Terry (2001) On the record. *Primary Care Management* 11(4) 26

Children (Leaving Care) Act 2000: chapter 35. London: The Stationery Office

Summary: this Act aims to implement the proposals of *Me, survive, out there?(1999).* It amends the *Children Act 1989*, providing for young people in care to move into independent living. A duty is placed on local authorities not only to assess and meet the needs of eligible young people, but also to assist those formerly in their care in respect of education, employment and training. The local authority has a duty to stay in contact with all these eligible care leavers, including eighteen to twentyone year olds. The Act also simplifies the financial support arrangements for young people. It enables local authorities to accommodate, support and advise those leaving care, and will avoid the situation that has formerly existed whereby care leavers were simply given money and left to fend for themselves.

Further reading:
Bateman, N. (2000) Welfare rights: October benefits revolution? *Community Care* 14 .12.2000 29

Department of Health (1999) *Me, survive, out there? New arrangements for young people living in and leaving care.* London: The Stationery Office

Piper, Mari (2000) *A care leaver's perspective.* London: Department of Health

Rickford, Frances (2000) Help is at hand. *Community Care* 5.7.2000 18-19

Madge, Nicola et al (2000) *Nine to thirteen: the forgotten years?* London: National Children's Bureau

Summary: this takes the view that whilst most children pass through the years from nine to thirteen without incident, this is a period of change from childhood to adolescence when problems may arise for the first time such as delinquency, substance abuse and sexual violence on the one hand, abuse and neglect on the other. The report argues for an increased focus on services for this age group since at this age, it is still possible to stop problems in their tracks.

Department of Health (2000) *Adopting changes: survey and inspection of local councils' adoption services.* London: The Stationery Office

Summary: the results of a national survey conducted by the Social Services Inspectorate, evaluating local councils' adoption services and designed to give a detailed picture of current practice in order to plan for change. The issues are:

- many councils have good adoption practice but in some councils there are children in need of adoptive families who are not found them

- the time taken to identify an adoption varies greatly, the whole process taking anything from six months to four and a half years. Some of these delays arise because of a lack of trained staff and some because of difficulties placing children who have medical problems, disabilities or emotional/behavioural difficulties. However, councils' policies, procedures and practice guidance are by no means universal or consistent; the report states the need to address ALL avoidable causes of delay

- the report also finds that potential adopters were put off by the delay in response in some cases and by the tone of response in others. For many, the whole process took far longer than they were led to expect

- 'post-adoption' services are underdeveloped in all areas

Department of Health (2000) *Adoption: a new approach.* London: The Stationery Office

Summary: a white paper that proposes speeding up the adoption process and putting the needs of children first by introducing new legislation and procedures. Amongst these proposals are an investment of £66.5 million over three years and a 40% increase in number of adoptions by 2004/5. Councils are to improve their adoption practices and ultimately achieve a 50% increase in numbers of children adopted. The supporting legislation provides for:

- an adoption register holding details of approved adoptive families and of children waiting for adoption

- a new legal framework for adoption allowances

- an independent review mechanism for assessing potential adopters
- for adoptees: access to information about their history
- the payment of court fees by councils once 'looked-after' children are adopted
- bringing the *Children Act 1989* and the *Adoption Act 1976* into line

There will also be a consultation for National Adoption Standards: aimed at all those involved in the adoption process this will clarify expectations, placing the needs of the child first.

Other proposals include: paid adoption leave for one parent of an adopted child; practice guidelines for councils; a range of powers to deal with councils that fail to provide a reasonable level of service; increased flexibility for courts in the family justice system in specialised adoption court centres.

Further reading:

Anon (2001) Adoption: a new approach. *Childright* no. 173 Jan/Feb 8-10

Rickford, F (2001) Good on paper. *Community Care* 1.2.2001 18-19

Adams, K. (2001) *Developing quality to protect children: SSI inspection of children's services, August 1999 - July 2000.* London: The Stationery Office

Summary: a report summarising the findings of thirty one local inspections of children's services following the Quality Protects initiative. It provides a starting point from which future improvements can be measured.

The quality of the services varied greatly from council to council although no single council was better or worse than the rest as they all had good and bad points. There was evidence that bodies such as education authorities and other health agencies were becoming increasingly involved in the planning and implementation of children's services and the importance of this was widely recognised. The Quality Protects programme was clearly being implemented, only some councils were further 'down the line' than others.

Specific problems were highlighted: in 6% of cases, children requiring protection were considered not to have been adequately safeguarded; this was brought to the attention of senior managers. Another problem was that training was judged to be low or insufficient in areas such as child protection, inter-agency work, assessment work and communicating with children. In many areas however the situation was seen to be improving.

Adoption and Children Act 2002: chapter 38. London: The Stationery Office

Summary: follows the white paper *Adoption: a new approach (2000)* and provides for an adoption service that makes the child's welfare paramount. Local authorities to be responsible for maintaining an adoption register and adoption support services. Other provisions include:

- regulation of local adoption agencies
- permits adoption by a single person as well as married or unmarried couples
- provides for a more rigorous approach to disclosing information about birth parents

- restrictions to the practice of bringing in children from overseas as well as advertising children (including on the internet) and restrictions to certain payments in connexion with this
- Secretary of State to establish a register to match children with adopters

The Act also amends the *Children Act 1989* including as follows:

- allows unmarried fathers to take on parental responsibility
- introduces guardianship as a way of giving permanence to those children not suitable for adoption
- local authorities to arrange advocacy services
- amends the definition 'harm to a child' to include their witnessing ill-treatment of others

Home Office (2003) *The Victoria Climbie inquiry report (cm5730)*. (chair Herbert Laming) London: The Stationery Office

Summary: in the last eleven months of her life in England Victoria Climbie was subjected to unprecedented abuse, the like of which had not been encountered or recorded before and which led to her death on 25th February 2002. The abuse continued in spite of her case being known to three housing authorities, four social services departments, two child protections teams of the Metropolitan Police and a centre managed by the NSPCC in the local authority areas of Haringey, Ealing and Brent. Because of suspected abuse Victoria was admitted twice to two different hospitals and still no one intervened for her protection. The report details breakdowns of management, communication and responsibilities, expressing abhorrence that whilst front-line staff were suspended, managers moved on and away from the situation. The report makes 108 recommendations including:

- establish a Children and Families Board chaired at cabinet level with ministerial representatives, and a National Agency for Children and Families,
- local authorities to replace their focus on completing bureaucratic targets with working towards "outcomes for people", ensuring clear lines of accountability in child protection
- establish Committees for Children and Families to oversee the work of local authorities, police, education and health services
- establish a Management for Services to Children and Families to ensure service delivery including the effectiveness of interagency working
- lines of communication should be improved as well as the quality of information exchanged and the way it is brought together for assessment
- Government to address where free exchange of information is inhibited by data protection and human rights legislation
- establish a National Children's Database, built up from entries by staff in any key service so as to build up a comprehensive picture of a child's current state and needs in any area
- local authorities to ensure that money allocated for child welfare really is spent on child welfare

- local authorities to take a lead in social regeneration and inclusion, moving away from self-serving activities that support the organisation rather than the public they're intended to serve

- as families are most likely to be together 'out-of-hours', professional services should be available then and NOT staffed by agency/locum workers

Consideration is also given to issues of race, education and practice documentation.

Further reading:

Bullock, R. (2003) Child protection post-Laming: the wider agenda. *Journal of Integrated Care* 11(5) 13-7

Chand, A. (2003) 'Race' and the Laming report on Victoria Climbie: lessons for interprofessional policy and practice. *Journal of Integrated Care* 11(4) 27-8

Cowan, J. (2003) Risk management, records and the Laming report. *Clinical Governance* 8(3) 271-77

Department for Education and Skills (2003) *The Government's response to the Health Committee's sixth report of session 2002-03 on the Victoria Climbie inquiry report (cm5992)*. London: The Stationery Office

House of Commons Health Committee (2003) *The Victoria Climbie Inquiry Report, Sixth Report of Session 2002-03 HC 570*. London: The Stationery Office

Hudson, B. (2004) Willing but able? *Community Care* 17.6.2004 36-7

Laming, Lord Herbert (2003) We owe it to Victoria's memory. *Community Care* 18.8.2003 40-41

Home Office (2003) *Safeguarding children: the joint Chief Inspectors' report on arrangements to safeguard children.* London: The Stationery Office

Summary: instigated by recommendations made in *Modernising social services (1998)*, the report is the result of a programme of inspections of safeguards for children contributed to by the inspectorates of HMs: Prisons, Crown Prosecution, Magistrates, Probation, Constabulary, and Social Services, the Office for Standards in Education and the CHI. Positive findings include:

- where children are identified as being at risk, they are protected from further harm

- where children are on the Child Protection register, social workers are working well with other agencies and overall, interagency work was good, with the ability to work flexibly a key to good relationships

Chief among the concerns were:

- the problem of recruiting and retaining qualified, experienced staff

- Area Child Protection Committees lack resources and authority

- with all their other commitments, local authorities don't always give priority to safeguarding children

- prison inspectors anxious about the welfare of young people in young offender institutions

- an inconsistent approach to protecting children from dangerous persons or offenders using MAPPPs i.e. Multi Agency Public Protection Panels

- certain service areas not well integrated into local service e.g. GPs, mental health services, independent schools

Department of Health, Home Office and Department for Education and Skills (2003) *Keeping children safe: the Government's response to the Victoria Climbie inquiry report and Joint Chief Inspectors' report Safeguarding children (cm5861).* London: The Stationery Office

Summary: written in response to the Victoria Climbie and other inquiries into incidents of child abuse as well as *Safeguarding children (2003)*. Whilst the basis of the *Children Act 1989* remains sound, systems fail because:

- frontline staff are under too much pressure and unsupported by their seniors
- management fail to take responsibility for their staff and services
- standards and priorities vary across the country
- Area Child Protection Committees lack resources and authority
- social services have problems with recruiting and retaining staff
- there is uncertainty about when and to whom to share information about a child

Incidence of abuse and death from abuse can be lowered by effective support and early intervention and needs: sound legislation; multi-agency team working with coordinated needs assessment and regular review; involving children and families in decision-making; adequate staff levels that are well-trained and strongly supported. Full details of proposed reforms appear in *Every child matters (2003)*.

Further reading:
Platt, D. (2003) *What to do if you're worried a child is being abused.* London: Department of Health

Department for Education and Skills (2003) *Every child matters.* London: DfES

Summary: a plan for reform based on what matters most in the eyes of children and young people i.e.: being healthy and staying safe, enjoying and achieving, making a positive contribution to society, and economic security. Improvements so far have included the Sure Start programme; full service extended schools schemes opening 'out-of-hours' and offering health and social care facilities; the *Young People's Fund;* investment in child and adolescent mental health services; initiatives to tackle homelessness and reform of the youth justice system. Proposals are based on:

- supporting parents with parenting funds, information and advice services, engaging parents in their child's development and progress
- early intervention and support: sharing information, establishing a common assessment framework, multi-agency teams working directly in schools, children's centres etc
- accountability and integration: directors of children's services to be accountable for local education and social services; appointment of a lead councillor for children; children's trusts to integrate the different key services within the local authority;

Local Safeguarding Children Boards to replace the Area Child Protection Committees; appointment of a Minister for Children and Young People and a Children's Commissioner to report yearly to Parliament and act as a children's champion

- workforce reform: improving skills and providing incentives; recruitment campaigns; flexible working and training, with core skills for all who work with children; leadership programme. All this supported by the Children's Workforce Unit and Sector Skills Council for Children and Young People's Services

Further reading:

Social Exclusion Unit (2003) *Raising the educational attainment of children in care.* London: SEU

Department for Education and Skills (2003) *Youth justice: the next steps.* London: DfES

House of Commons Work and Pensions Committee (2004) *Child poverty in the UK.* London: The Stationery Office

Summary: looks at the impact of the Government's child poverty reduction strategy. Reports success and the conviction that the goal of reducing child poverty by 25% by the end of 2004 will be reached. A different approach will be needed for the 2010 goal to succeed. This should focus on particular social groups with improvements in health, education and transport services as well as affordable child care. The report recommends increasing financial support by £10 per week for poorest children and goes on to make another 21 specific recommendations such as:

- ear marked funds for provision of school clothing and school meals
- payments of 'development grants' for key stages in a child's life
- sustain commitment to keep child benefit at real value
- reconsider requiring single parents to be in work as a condition of receiving benefit
- recruit older people into the childcare workforce
- research into the factors influencing stable parenting and life chances
- develop and expand the role of the social fund

Further reading:

Adelman, L. Middleton, S. and Ashworth, K. (2003) *Britain's poorest children: severe and persistent and social exclusion.* London: Save the Children

Howard, M. (2001) *Paying the price: carers, poverty and social exclusion.* London: Child Poverty Action Group

Department of Education and Skills and Department of Health (2004) *National service framework for children, young people and maternity services.* London: Department of Health

Summary: a detailed and comprehensive, evidence-based set of standards to support needs-led child-centred services (for maternity services see Midwifery chapter). The children and young component represents a part of the *Change for children - every child matters* programme that is committed to supporting children: to be healthy and safe, to enjoy life, to make a contribution and find economic stability. Eleven standards are arranged as follows:

1. health promotion, disease prevention and early intervention with problems
2. supporting parents
3. child and family-centred services
4. adolescence
5. safeguarding the welfare of children and young people
6. care of sick children and young people
7. children and young people in hospital
8. children and young people with disabilities and complex needs
9. mental health
10. medicines
11. maternity services

Further reading:
Hainsworth, T. (2004) The NSF for children, young people and maternity services. *Nursing Times* 100(40) 28-30

Children Act 2004: chapter 31. London: The Stationery Office

Summary: written in the light of green paper *Every child matters (2003)* and the *Victoria Climbie inquiry (2002)* the Act:

- provides for a Children's Commissioner to represent children and promote their interests and safety in England
- commits local authorities to arrange for key agencies to cooperate to improve the welfare of children and young people
- requires children's services authorities to produce a Children and Young People's Plan
- makes key agencies responsible for ensuring children's welfare and safety
- establishes statutory Local Safeguarding Children Boards to replace the non-statutory Area Child Protection Committees
- provides for the creation of a Children and Young People's Database
- provides for English local authorities to appoint a Director of Children's Services to stand accountable for local authorities' education and social services to children
- creates an integrated inspection framework so that inspections may cover and review all services provided to children (education, social, health, housing etc)
- provides for similar structures and appointments in Wales

Other provisions include:

- stronger notification arrangements in private fostering
- simplifying the registration of child minder and day care providers
- local authorities to promote educational achievements of children in care
- limit the grounds by which hitting a child may be seen as reasonable punishment
- before deciding on services to a child in need, local authorities to ascertain and give consideration to the child's wishes

Further reading:

Kelley, N. (2004) Child's play. *Community care* 1.7.04 34-5

Whitfield, L. (2004) Toeing the line. *Health Service Journal* 114(5903) 28-9

Supplementary reading:

Audit Commission (2000) *Children in mind: child and adolescent mental health services.* London: Audit Commission

Bellamy, C. (2002) *The state of the world's children 2003.* New York: UNICEF

Department for Education and Skills and Department of Health (2004) *Children's and maternity services information strategy.* London: Department of Health

Department of Education and Department of Health (1994) *The education of sick children.* London: HMSO

Department of Health (2003) F*ostering services: national minimum standards; fostering services regulations.* London: The Stationery Office

Department of Health (1999) *Me, survive, out there? New arrangements for young people living in and leaving care.* London: The Stationery Office

Department of Health (2003) *Neonatal intensive care review.* London: Department of Health

Department of Health (2001) *The Children Act report 2000.* London: The Stationery Office

Department of Social Services (1988) *Report of the inquiry into child abuse in Cleveland 1987.* (chair Elizabeth Butler-Sloss) London: HMSO

Hall, David M. B. (ed) (2003) *Health for all children. 4th ed.* Oxford: Oxford University Press

Hogg, Christine (1998) *Child friendly primary health care.* London: Action for Sick Children

McHaffie, H. E. et al (1999) Withholding / withdrawing treatment from neonates: legislation and official guidelines across Europe. *Journal of Medical Ethics* 25(6) 440-446

NHS Estates (2003) *Improving the patient experience: friendly health care environments for children and young people.* London: Department of Health

NHS Executive (1996) *Child health in the community: a guide to good practice.* London: Department of Health

O'Neale, V. (2000) *Excellence not excuses: inspection of services for ethnic minority children and families.* London: The Stationery Office

Performance and Innovation Unit (2000) *Prime Minister's review: adoption: issued for consultation.* London: Cabinet Office: PIU

Platt, D. (2001) *Access to education for children and young people with medical needs.* London: Department of Health

Royal College of Paediatrics and Child Health and the Joint British Advisory Committee on Children's Nursing (1996) *Developing roles of nurses in clinical child health.* London: Royal College of Paediatrics and Child Health

Slater, Mary (1993) *Health for all our children: achieving appropriate healthcare for black and ethnic minority children.* London: Action for Sick Children

Stoate, H and Jones, B. (2003) *All's well that starts well: a strategy for children's health.* London: Fabian Society

Walker, Alison (1996) *Young carers and their families: a survey carried out by the Social Survey Division of the ONS on behalf of the Department of Health.* London: The Stationery Office

8 Mental Health

Department of Health (1983) *Mental Health Act 1983: chapter 20.*
London: HMSO

Summary: amends some of the provisions of the 1959 Act. Coverage includes: access to Mental Health Tribunals; participation of the whole multidisciplinary team (nurses, psychiatrists, psychologists, social workers) in decisions on treatment and detention; consent to treatment; mentally disordered offenders; community and informal psychiatric care.

Further reading:
Dimond, Bridget (1984) The Mental Health Act 1983. *Community Care* 23.2.1984 23-6

Killen, S. (1983) Nurses and the Mental Health Act. *Nursing Times* 79(37) 44-48

Mawson, D. (1986) Seeking informed consent...1983 Mental Health Act. *Nursing Times* 82(6) 52-53

Webster, L. Dean, C. and Kessel, N. (1987) Effect of the 1983 Mental Health Act on the management of psychiatric patients. *British Medical Journal* 295(6612) 1529-32

Department of Health (1994) *The health of the nation key area handbook: mental illness. 2nd ed.* London: HMSO.

Summary: expands on the targets in *The health of the nation (1992)* white paper. Recommends improving the health of the mentally ill and reducing suicide rates. Looks at changes in services, treatment methods and settings.

Further reading:
Murdock, D. (1995) Redefining the targets for mental illness. *Nursing Standard* 10(49) 28-30

House of Commons Health Committee (1994) *Better off in the community?: the care of people who are seriously mentally ill: 1st report.* London: HMSO

Summary: this report looks at the transition from institutionalised to community care and the closure of institutions. Particular areas covered are: the care programme approach (CPA); safety and security of the public in relation to care in the community of mentally ill patients; the homeless mentally ill; responsibilities of institutionalised care settings; future service patterns to be in place by the year 2000; interdepartmental cooperation between health and social services and closer monitoring of existing community care systems for the mentally ill.

Audit Commission (1994) *Finding a place: a review of mental health services for adults.* London: HMSO

Summary: this report concentrates on services provided for adults with mental health problems. It describes how historically policy has shifted from care in large psychiatric hospitals to care in the community. Concerns over the slow implementation of community care policy are discussed along with the allocation of resources, and the patchy implementation of the care programme approach. The report concludes that the way forward involves strengthening leadership and management, and identifies the main challenges as:

- the correct targeting and management of the service
- reviewing the pattern of resource distribution

The consequences for the commissioning authorities and different agencies is then examined

Further reading
Shepherd, G. (1995) Finding a place: a review of mental health services for adults. *Journal of Mental Health* 4(1) 9-16

Department of Health (1995) *Mental Health (Patients in the Community) Act 1995: chapter 52.* London: HMSO

Summary: this Act is concerned with the care and supervision of patients with mental disorders after their discharge from hospital. It states the criteria under which health authorities may apply for a supervision order, e.g. where a patient may still be considered to be a risk to the safety of himself or others. It updates the 1983 Act on areas such as the role of medical practitioners, and patients' leave of absence from hospital.

Further reading:
Coffey, M. (1996) Supervised discharge...Mental Health Act 1995. *Nursing Times* 92(26) 50-3

Department of Health (1996) *Building bridges: a guide to inter-agency working for the care and protection of severely mentally ill people.* London: HMSO

Summary: this report aims to encourage inter-agency working. Aimed at mental health professionals, managers and purchasers it provides information about the care programme approach, the current legislative framework and discusses issues such as client confidentiality and information sharing. The report also outlines the roles of the various agencies involved and how they should best work together. There is information about auditing services as well as continuing education and training.

Sheppard, David (1996) *Learning the lessons: mental health inquiry reports published in England and Wales between 1969 and 1996 and their recommendations for improving practice. 2nd ed* London: Zeto Trust

Summary: collation of inquiry reports about homicides involving mental health patients. This second edition documents fifty four independent inquiries and over three hundred recommendations. The first half of the publication lists each inquiry with details of the incident and the terms of reference of the inquiry. The second half contains a list of the various recommendations arranged chronologically by subject.

Thornicroft, G. and Strathdee, G. (1996) *Commissioning mental health services.* London: HMSO

Summary: for those involved in purchasing and commissioning mental health services, this report gives information about good practice, current areas of debate and details of population-based service planning. Four sections cover:
- the national policy framework within which commissioning takes place
- the perspectives of purchasers and commissioners
- the commissioning process from the provider's perspective
- the implementation of policy

Department of Health (1997) *The patient's charter: mental health services.* London: HMSO

Summary: a booklet that summarises the principles of the *Patient's charter (1991)* then outlines patients' rights in the context of mental health. Areas covered include confidentiality, the care programme approach, discharge from hospital and an explanation of the *Mental Health Act 1983.* A list of addresses covers organisations concerned with mental health care.

Department of Health (1997) *Developing partnerships in mental health (cm3555).* London: The Stationery Office

Summary: a green paper that describes the government's commitment to developing partnerships in the care of people with severe mental illness. The document emphasises the importance of integrating the work of statutory, voluntary and independent agencies to provide a seamless mental health service.

It concludes with options for structural changes and seeks views from interested parties on which approaches would be the most effective. These options are:
- establishing a new mental health and social care authority
- establishing either the health authority or local authority as a single agency
- combining the health and local authorities to create a joint health and social care body
- allowing health and local authorities to delegate functions and responsibilities to each other

Further reading
Ashman, M. (1997) Green, green grass of change. *Mental Health Nursing* 17(2) 4-5

Mental Health Act Commission and Sainsbury Centre (1997) *The national visit: a one-day visit to 309 acute psychiatric wards by the Mental Health Act Commission in collaboration with the Sainsbury Centre for Mental Health*. London: Sainsbury Centre for Mental Health

Summary: a snapshot view of acute inpatient facilities that looked in particular at detained patients who were absent without leave, the care of women patients, and nursing staff. Findings include:

- with the emphasis on care in the community, inpatient care has been neglected
- inpatient care involves a heavy workload and staff were having difficulty ensuring leave was properly authorised
- many women have to share facilities with men, 3% even sleeping in the same area; half the wards reported problems of sexual harassment
- although staffing is adequate, nurses were not always in contact with patients and lacked the skills and support needed to communicate effectively with patients who had severe illnesses such as schizophrenia and manic-depression

The report recommends viewing inpatient and community psychiatric care as an integrated whole, improving management and leadership; updating nurses skills through training and addressing the issue of safety for women patients.

Firth, Malcolm and Kerfoot, Michael (1997) *Voices in partnership: involving users and carers in commissioning and delivering mental health services*. London: The Stationery Office

Summary: this report outlines the challenges to user and carer participation in the development of NHS services for mental health and makes recommendations as to how they are addressed. The report is based on research carried out in 1994-96 on adults using mental health services and their adult carers. The effects of recent legislation, the role of users and carers in service planning and delivery and sources of conflict are considered. Recommendations are made for the way forward. These include employment of salaried workers, training as care/service professionals, mainstream funding and the wider development of professional advocacy for users and carers.

Department of Health (1998) *Tackling drugs to build a better Britain: the government's ten year strategy for tackling drug misuse*. London: The Stationery Office

Summary: this aims to take a new, long-term approach to the drugs issue. The strategy is based on an extensive review by the UK anti-drugs coordinator, Keith Halliwell, who contributes to the document.

The main elements are:

- inform and educate young people about drugs

- help drug misusing offenders to tackle their drug problems and thereby reduce the levels of crime

- increase the participation of drug misusers, including prisoners, in drug treatment programmes

- reduce the availability of drugs

Each element of the strategy relies on statutory, voluntary and private sectors working in partnership, and for there being a rigorous assessment of the effectiveness of implementing the strategy, using research, audit and consultation.

Further reading:

Farrell, M. and Strang, J. (1998) Britain's new strategy for tackling drugs misuse shows a welcome emphasis on evidence. *British Medical Journal* 316(142) 1399-400

Department of Health (1998) *Modernising mental health services: safe, sound and supportive*. London: Department of Health

Summary: as part of the Government's modernisation of the NHS, this reviews the current state of mental health, noting the high level of suicide in young people as well as the link between severe mental illness and violence. Proposals for improvement include:

- creating a needs-led service that will also protect the public

- full access to service including a 24-hour crisis service

- supporting families and carers as well as patients

- establishing integrated care by working with agencies in education, housing and employment

- under guidance from NICE, ensuring service is efficient and cost effective

The Government plans to commit £700 million to improvements over three years. These will include the provision of extra beds and better outreach services. Primary care groups will work closely with specialist teams to integrate planning and delivery. Secure hospitals will be improved. Performance will be monitored through new assessment frameworks for health and social care, and a new national service framework for mental health will determine service models and standards (see below).

Further reading:

Jackson, Catherine (1999) Gold blend. *Mental Health Care* 2(6) 190-1

McFadyen, J.A. (1999) Modernising mental health services: the right ACT for the wrong reason? *British Journal of Health Care Management* 5(1) 28-34

Royal College of Nursing (1999) *RCN mental health nursing strategy*. London: RCN

Scott, Helen (1998) Review of mental health law must be courageous. *British Journal of Nursing* 7(19) 1138

Department of Health (1998) *Mental Health Act 1983: memorandum on parts I to IV, VIII and X.* London: The Stationery Office

Summary: this is intended as guidance for mental health workers on implementing the 1983 Act. It covers the sections which deal with patient admission, supervised discharge, remand, consent to treatment and detention under the Act. It also defines and clarifies some of the terms used in the Act and is recommended to be read in conjunction with the new *Code of practice (1999)*.

Department of Health (1999) *Code of practice: Mental Health Act 1983.* London: The Stationery Office

Summary: for use by all health professionals in the field of mental health as well as the police and social services. This code gives guidance on how the 1983 Act should be applied in the light of new law and terminology. It highlights the rights of individuals under the *European Convention on Human Rights (1978)* and encourages the use of the new Care Programme Approach in mental health services. The code also stresses the importance of communication with patients, confidentiality and giving information to patients and their relatives.

Further reading:

Bluglass, Robert (1983) *A guide to the Mental Health Act 1983.* Edinburgh: Churchill Livingstone

Dolan, Bridget and Powell, Debra (2001) *The point of law: the Mental Health Act explained.* London: The Stationery Office

Department of Health (1999) *Safer services: national confidential inquiry into suicide and homicide by people with mental illness.* (chair Louis Appleby) London: Department of Health

Summary: report commissioned to collect data on mental health patients in England and Wales who have committed suicide or homicide, and to recommend health policy to reduce the risks of such incidents in the future. The findings consider factors such as: last contact with mental health services; prevention; in-patient and post-discharge; homelessness; non-compliance with treatment; previous violent offences; drug and alcohol misuse and dependence and ethnic groups. Key findings include:

- 24% of suicide cases were in contact with mental health services during the previous year, and the inquiry believes that many are not inevitable but preventable through improved services to reduce risk
- 8% of convicted homicides were in contact with mental health services in the previous year and 14% at some time, mostly for substance dependence or personality disorder rather than mental illness, but these cases were less preventable than the suicides
- the majority of homicides have a history of violence and substance misuse

Among the recommendations for improving mental health services are:

- regular staff training concentrating on high risk groups and substance misuse
- to ensure that all relevant information reaches every agency involved, streamlined

documentation in the form of 'patient passports' that will record mental health history and previous violent offences

- new 'atypical' drug treatment to be used where possible to reduce risk of side effects; non-compliance information to be better documented
- health authorities to have a better policy for those who are disengaged from services, including methods of outreach
- measures to prevent in-patient suicides such as increased monitoring and the removal of structures which could be used for hanging
- better follow-up after discharge in at-risk cases, giving help with finding accommodation
- use of mental health legislation in cases of high risk or non-compliance
- highest level of care under the care programme approach (CPA)

Finally, the Committee believes that the Department of Health should re-evaluate the system of local inquiries into cases: the present system often engenders a 'culture of blame' against staff and therefore do not always produce worthwhile results.

Standing Nursing and Midwifery Advisory Committee (1999) *Mental health nursing: "addressing acute concerns".* (chair Tony Bell) London: Department of Health

Summary: with the shift from hospital to community care in recent years, the report finds that in spite of the severity of patients' illnesses and the complexity of their needs, acute mental health care has deteriorated. Issues include:

- staffing: there is poor clinical leadership; inadequate education and training; insufficient staff numbers with problems of recruitment and retention; and a lack of support from other professional groups
- safety: women and other vulnerable groups have little privacy and are vulnerable to assault and sexual abuse; violence and aggression is also a problem for staff
- race: the needs of minority groups are not recognised and staff themselves are subject to racial discrimination
- health policy: mental health nurses are not practicing evidence-based care or involving users and carers in planning, practising and evaluating care

Recommendations are directed at various agencies and include:

- NHS executive to develop evidence-based guidelines for acute mental health care
- Chief Nursing Officers to promote clinical leadership and the recognition of acute care as a worthwhile career
- education: service and education providers to collaborate to produce programmes in: acute care, assessment, risk assessment, involving users, the management of violence, and interventions including medication and therapies
- research is needed to improve the evidence base in acute care, the therapeutic culture and liaison nursing

- employers to develop formal methods of patient assessment; involve users and carers; make better use of liaison nurses in casualty departments; develop clinical leadership; promote nurse consultant posts; promote staff and patient safety; consider needs of minority groups and racial discrimination within staffing structures

Department of Health (1999) *National service framework for mental health: modern standards and service models.* London: Department of Health

Summary: building on the principles outlined in *Modernising mental health services (1998),* this framework establishes standards and models of service delivery. For the first time, milestones and performance indicators are set, against which progress can be measured. Aimed at the adult population to age sixty five, the framework covers five areas:

- mental health promotion
- primary care
- access to services
- effective care for those with severe mental illness, and the prevention of suicide
- support for carers

Further reading:
Tyrer, P. (1999) The national service framework: a scaffold for mental health. *British Medical Journal* 319(7216) 1017-8

Thornicroft, G. (2000) National service framework for mental health. *Psychiatric Bulletin* 24(6) 203-6

Faculty of Health, University of Central Lancashire (1999) *Nursing in secure environments.* London: United Kingdom Central Council for Nursing, Midwifery and Health Visiting

Summary: a commissioned study that aims to present a picture of what is expected of nurses in secure environments in order to create an action plan. The study looked at nursing in secure hospitals and in prisons where many issues arise with their responsibility for maintaining security as well as giving care. The study also found that working in 'closed' institutions led to difficulties with developing practice and sustaining relationships. Recommendations cover education, the evidence base, standards and competencies, clinical supervision, managing violence and challenging behaviour as well as cultural and gender issues.

Further reading:
Polczyk-Przybyla, M. and Gournay, Kevin (1999) Psychiatric nursing in prison: the state of the art? *Journal of Advanced Nursing* 30(4) 893-900

Audit Commission (2000) *Forget me not: mental health services for older people.* London: Audit Commission (see Chapter 7. Older People)

Mental Health Foundation (2000) *Strategies for living: a report of user-led research into people's strategies for living with mental distress.* London: MHF

Summary: 76 people were interviewed to find out how they coped with mental illness or distress; what treatments were helpful - e.g. medication or 'talking therapies', and what strategies they used to help themselves such as exercise, creative activities etc. This was a three-year study whose aims were to help other sufferers by publicising these strategies, promoting a holistic approach to mental health care, and encouraging user-led research in mental health. Participants were chosen on the basis of their experience of different therapies, ethnic origin, age and geographic location, with an almost equal ratio of men to women. Also involved were people with severe mental health problems. As regards treatments and strategies for coping, variety seems to be key, but the study also gives valuable insight into users' perceptions of mental health services as well as the effect of living with the stigma of mental illness.

Department of Health (2000) *Reforming the Mental Health Act. Part 1: the new legal framework (cm5016-I); part 2: high risk patients (cm5016-II)* London: The Stationery Office

Summary: this two-part white paper applies to mental health care in England only.

Part 1: the new legal framework deals with the detention of the small minority of people with a mental illness who present a risk to themselves and others. A new framework is needed effectively to detain patients without contravening the *Human Rights Act 1998*.

- established criteria must be met before detention in each case, the decision to detain made by three mental health professionals
- the initial period of detention is to be no more than 28 days before being assessed by the Mental Health Tribunal who may authorise a further six or twelve months during which a specific care plan must be followed
- in some cases compulsory powers may be applied to patients cared for in the community: for instance in administering medication or attending day care
- rights and safeguards: patients and their relatives are to be informed of the law under which they are being treated; they may request a review of the Mental Health Tribunal Order; they must have the opportunity to take free legal and advocacy advice; they may be involved in treatment plans when social and cultural backgrounds should be considered
- a specialist in child mental health must be involved in treatment plans for children
- a new Commission for Mental Health will protect patients' interests, oversee the use of legislation, ensure training needs are met and must be consulted when patients are unable to give consent to treatment and when ECT and psychosurgery are recommended as treatments

Part 2: high risk patients sets policy in the light of Government's priority to protect the safety of the public. It details assessment criteria and care of detainees. Two categories are named: those who present a danger to themselves and those who are a danger to others.

- health and social care workers to act in cooperation with agencies such as the police, the courts and prison and probation services, acting in consideration of legislation such as the *Criminal Justice Act 2000*
- care plans to emphasise therapeutic treatment as well as detention
- for the dangerous and severely personality disordered (DSPD) group, pilot schemes run in 2001 may result in new powers for mental health practitioners, and lead to the creation of specific accommodation in prisons, hospitals and community hostels. A specialist team will decide whether DSPD status applies and where there is a criminal conviction, courts can choose between a prison sentence, a care and treatment order, a restriction order or a hospital and limitation direction
- there will be more sharing of information between health and social care and law enforcement services, particularly in cases of violent and sexual crimes. Relevant departments to be alerted when a patient or offender leaves detention or moves between NHS and prison services
- Mental Health Tribunals can set conditions on a patient's discharge and in some cases, recall them to detention

Further reading:

Dimond, B. (2001) Reform of mental health law must not be rushed. *British Journal of Nursing* 10(2) 69

Donnelly, L. (2001) A tough nut to crack. Health Service Journal 111(5737) 11-12

Grounds, A. (2001) Reforming the Mental Health Act. *British Journal of Psychiatry* 179 387-9

Jackson, C. (2001) Law and disordered. *Mental Health and Learning Disabilities Care* 4(6) 184-5

Department of Health (2002) *National suicide prevention strategy for England.* London: Department of Health

Summary: part of the *Saving lives (1999)* target to reduce suicide deaths by 20% in 2010. The 'on-going', 'evolving' strategy proposes six goals:

- reducing risk in high risk groups: projects targeting young men's mental health; monitoring non-fatal self harm and supporting local services management of risk with *12 points to a safer service*
- improve public mental health generally: looking at issues such as housing and unemployment, managing substance misuse in young men who self-harm
- make suicide less easy to achieve: promoting safer prescribing and looking at 'hotspots' such as railways and bridges
- involving the media: encourage responsible reporting and how suicide is represented in the press etc
- promote and disseminate research
- improve monitoring processes

Department of Health (2002) *Developing services for carers and families of people with mental illness.* London: Department of Health

Summary: aimed at local mental health services to read alongside Standard Six of the NSF: *Caring for carers*, the report focuses on carers of people with severe mental illness and who are on the Care Programme Approach. Support is vital, for the impact of mental illness on the carer can be similar to the sufferer in terms of affecting work, education, finances and social life as well as their own physical and emotional health. Carers are also vital as the first point of contact at the onset of illness. Service providers should:

- recognise the valuable role of carers and the stress they are under
- provide timely support or help if they can no longer carry on
- involve carers in planning and developing future services

Support should include: information and advice, including advocacy, breaks and access to interventions such as family therapy. Services should be based on four principles: 1) positive and inclusive 2) flexible and needs-led 3) accessible and responsive and 4) integrated and coordinated. Chapters follow on commissioning services; identifying and assessing carers; carers who are young people or from minority ethnic groups and the work of Carer Support Services.

Department of Health (2002) *Women's mental health: into the mainstream: strategic development of mental health care for women.* London: Department of Health

Summary: the *NHS plan (2000), Modernising mental health services (1998)* and the *Mental health NSF (1999)* all show a commitment to reduce inequalities in health and create a service that is responsive to the needs of its users. Mental illness is equally prevalent in men and women, but the way illness presents differs between them and services are not geared to respond. Women are susceptible to mental illness because of poverty, the stress of caring and parenting, lower employment levels and experience of violence and abuse. Particularly vulnerable are women from minority social groups such as offenders, substance abusers, prostitutes and so on. Recommendations include:

- women should be involved in care decisions as well as overall service planning
- there should be strong links with voluntary organisations with "robust commissioning arrangements" to ensure their financial stability
- the evidence base about women's mental health is limited: gender should be incorporated into research, and audit and evaluation processes
- women need to feel safe: they should have access to female staff and women-only facilities as well as support for them as parents through childcare facilities etc
- staff training needs to include an understanding of women's issues as well as addressing specifics such as abuse, violence and self-harm
- assessment and care must include consideration of socioeconomic factors in a woman's life, as well as dual diagnosis with substance abuse, risk assessment, physical health etc

Chapters follow on caring for women in community and acute settings and caring for specific groups such as women with experience of violence and abuse, with personality disorders and specific problems such as post-natal depression. This is a consultation document; *Mainstreaming gender and women's mental health (2003)* gives specific guidance to mental health and primary care trusts, strategic health authorities, local implementation teams and professional organisations.

Further reading:

Department of Health (2003) *Mainstreaming gender and women's mental health: implementation guidance.* London: Department of Health

The Women's Unit, Cabinet Office (1999) *Living without fear: an integrated approach to tackling violence against women.* London: Cabinet Office

Department of Health (2002) *The journey to recovery: the Government's vision for mental health care.* London: Department of Health

Summary: summarises the history of mental health care and the remedies for past problems in the form of *Modernising mental health services (1998)*, the *NSF for mental health (1999)*, plans to reform mental health legislation and the Care Programme Approach. Progress and plans include:

- change has been achieved through closer working with social services; in future, care trusts will be a merger of health and social services, integrating hospital and community care. New services will be tailored to meet local needs, paying particular attention to women's mental health, support for carers, personality disorders and collaboration with the criminal justice system
- the National Institute of Mental Health England has been established to support research, and improve and disseminate the evidence-base of effective treatments and therapies (see *Cases for change*)
- particular emphasis should be paid to staff recruitment, retention and training. Staff should be employed who reflect the communities they serve; issues of culture and race will be an integral part of pre-qualifying training for all mental health workers
- in the long term services will focus on recovery, with sufferers returning fully into society. Services to consider basic human needs, the need for social networks and friends, and removing the stigma of mental illness by changing society's attitude to it

National Institute for Mental Health England (2003) *Cases for change.* London: NIMHE

Summary: based on the best available evidence, these are ten booklets for frontline staff that aim to bring a summary of all the key issues associated with recent policy changes. Subjects include: partnership working, forensic services, user involvement and primary care.

National Institute for Mental Health England (2003) *Inside outside: improving mental health services for black and minority communities in England.* London: NIMHE

Summary: the lives of the 6.4 million people from different ethnic groups in England are subjected to discrimination and disadvantage, especially in health, with poorer health status, lower life expectancy and problems of access to care. The report refers to the *Race Relations (Amendment) Act 2000* requiring all public bodies to eliminate discrimination, promote equal opportunities and good relations between different racial groups. Within the mental health field, issues of ethnicity are invariably marginalised, the report aims to reduce marginalisation and discrimination looking in particular at three areas:

1. Inequalities in mental health service experience and outcome: there is a need for accountability and ownership of the needs of own community, with local implementation teams ensuring groups are represented and involved in decision-making. Clinical governance should be used as a mechanism to ensure high standards and improvement in services. Working methods should be adaptable to cultural needs, with collaboration with the voluntary sector. There is a need for interpreting services, good data gathering, and a willingness to tackle racism within organisations themselves. The report suggests target setting in four areas: primary care, care pathways, assessment and specialist services.

2. The cultural capability of the workforce: this looks at recruiting and supporting a multi-cultural workforce, and bringing 'cultural competencies' into education and training programmes.

3. Engaging the whole community: this suggests engaging Community Development Workers to help with organisational development, leadership, local concerns, developing local services, opportunities for education and training, and finding finance.

Department of Health (2004) *Draft Mental Health Bill (cm6305 - II).* London: The Stationery Office

Summary: redefines the legal framework for treating people with a mental disorder without their consent, almost completely replacing the *Mental Health Act 1983* (see above). The Secretary of State will issue a code of practice for using treatment under 'formal powers', with decisions and procedures following three stages: examination, assessment and treatment with further assessment if necessary. A first code will be for civilian patients, and a second for offenders coming through the criminal justice system. Although wherever possible patients are treated without compulsion, the 'curtailing of liberty' is to be managed in a way compatible with the European Convention on Human Rights. Before using formal powers, requirements include:

- consultation with people who know the patient; a new advocacy service is to be made available

- notification of certain persons and written records of decisions

- mental health tribunals (or in the case of mentally ill offenders, the courts) to make sure that treatment is scrutinised independently. They will authorise treatment under formal powers based on needs assessment and personal care plans

- treatment under formal powers may take place in the community as well as in hospital

- there are special safeguards for children under 16

The Bill would also provide for:

- administering treatments such as ECT and psychosurgery
- powers - including for the police - to enter property and detain patients for up to 72 hours
- support and representation for patients
- the extension of the functions of CHAI to replace the work of the Mental Health Act Commission
- dealing with offences such as obstruction, forgery, ill-treatment and wilful neglect

Further reading:

Daw, R. and Stone D. (2003) Winning hearts and minds. *Open Mind* Nov-Dec (124) 7

Gillen, S. (2004) Issue of detention remains a worry after the Mental Health Bill is redrawn. *Community Care* (1540) 16-7

National Institute for Mental Health England (2004) *Organising and delivering psychological therapies.* London: Department of Health

Summary: current services are patchy and inadequate in spite of convincing evidence of their effectiveness in treating mental health problems. Recommendations include:

- improvements in access
- services to provide more information about what therapies are available and how they may be accessed
- compose care pathways for the different problems and diseases
- address needs of particular groups such as older people and ethnic minority
- training for mental health professionals should be managed regionally on the basis of local needs assessment
- a Psychological Therapies Management Committee should oversee the service, making sure it is delivering evidence-based practice that is safe and appropriate and regularly audited

Office of the Deputy Prime Minister (2004) *Mental health and social exclusion: a Social Exclusion Unit report.* Wetherby: Office of the Deputy Prime Minister

Summary: people with mental health problems are invariably forced out onto the margins of society, losing friends, home and work, often with very little hope of reintegrating fully because of the stigma associated with mental illness. Suicide is common and the cost to the Government overall is high with more people in England claiming sickness benefit for illness than currently claiming Jobseekers Allowance. The causes of exclusion include: stigma, low expectations, lack of support in returning to work; barriers to integrating back into the community and racial discrimination. Especially vulnerable groups are young men, parents and those with complex needs. The report notes the progress that has been achieved via the NSF, the *Disability Discrimination Act 1995*, and the Pathways to Work pilot schemes. Points for action involve:

- a programme to dispel negative attitudes
- the role of health and social care
- employment
- supporting families and communities
- access to basics such as housing, transport, money advice etc
- target-setting to increase employment rates of people with disabilities, to reduce deaths from suicide and reduce child poverty

Robbins, D. for Social Services Inspectorate (2004) *Treated as people: an overview of mental health services from a social care perspective, 2003-4.* London: Department of Health

Summary: current policy requires that people with mental health problems receive timely and effective care and that they be seen in their whole, social context - not excluded because of the stigma of mental illness. Because of the requirement for joint agency (health and social care) working, this is the last time a report will cover social care on its own. Key findings include:

- the direct payments scheme is poorly developed
- the pressure of organisational change diverts attention away from the purpose of the service to deliver care
- local implementation teams report good progress as a result of the NSF, especially about working with carers. Services for ethnic minority users fall behind however
- whilst there are many isolated instances of good social care, failure to coordinate with other agencies means that social exclusion remains
- employment and accommodation services are good as they go, but insufficient to meet demand
- overall, clients want to be listened to and supported in the context of their lives
- increasingly (in England heading for 86% of all councils), social care is delivered within teams that include health services and are based on formal partnership arrangements

Supplementary Reading

Charlwood, P. et al (eds) (1999) *Health outcome indicators: severe mental illness: report of a working group to the Department of Health.* Oxford: National Centre for Health Outcomes Development

Clark, S. (2004) *Acute inpatient mental health care: education, training and continuing professional development for all.* London: Department of Health

Clinical Standards Advisory Group (1995) *Schizophrenia: volume 2: protocol for assessing services for people with a severe mental illness.* London: HMSO

Cohen, A. et al (2004) *The primary care guide to managing sever mental illness.* London: The Sainsbury Centre for Mental Health

Department of Health (1992) *Review of health and social services for mentally disordered offenders and others requiring similar services (cm2088).* (chair J.L. Reed) London: HMSO

Department of Health (1996) *Building bridges: a guide to arrangements for inter-agency working for the care and protection of severely mentally ill people: the health of the nation.* London: HMSO

Department of Health (2002) *Community mental health teams: policy implementation guide.* London: Department of Health

Department of Health (2003) *Fast-forwarding primary care mental health: 'gateway workers'.* London: Department of Health

Department of Health (2003) *Fast-forwarding primary care mental health: graduate primary care mental health workers: best practice guidance.* London: Department of Health

Department of Health (2001) *The mental health policy implementation guide.* London: Department of Health

Department of Health (2004) *The mental health policy implementation guide: adult acute inpatient care provision.* London: Department of Health

Department of Health (2004) *The mental health policy implementation guide: developing positive practice to support the safe and therapeutic management of aggression and violence in mental health inpatient settings.* London: Department of Health

Department of Health (2003) *The mental health policy implementation guide: dual diagnosis good practice guide.* London: Department of Health

Department of Health (2002) *The mental health policy implementation guide: national minimum standards for general adult services in psychiatric intensive care units and low secure environments.* London: Department of Health

Department of Health (2003) *The mental health policy implementation guide: support, time and recovery workers.* London: Department of Health

Department of Health (2003) *Personality disorder no longer a diagnosis of exclusion: policy implementation guidance for the development of services for people with personality disorder.* London: Department of Health

Department of Health (1996) *The spectrum of care: local services for people with mental health problems.* London: Department of Health

Echlin, R. (1995) *Partners in change: care planning in mental health services.* London: King's Fund

Lord Chancellor's Department (1999) *Making decisions: the government's proposals for making decisions on behalf of mentally incapacitated adults: a report issued in the light of the consultation paper "Who decides" (1997).* London: The Stationery Office

McCulloch, A. Warner, L. and Villeneau, L. (2000) *Taking your partners: using opportunities for inter-agency partnership in mental health.* London: Sainsbury Centre for Mental Health

Mental Health Foundation (1994) *Creating community care: report of the Mental Health Foundation inquiry into community care of people with severe mental illness.* London: Mental Health Foundation

Mental Health Foundation (2000) *Pull yourself together!: a survey of the stigma and discrimination faced by people who experience mental distress.* London: MHF

NHS Executive (1996) *NHS psychotherapy services in England: a review of strategic policy.* London: Department of Health

NHS Executive (1996) *24-hour nursed care for people with severe and enduring mental illness.* London: Department of Health

Royal College of Psychiatrists (1996) *Report of the confidential inquiry into homicides and suicides by mentally ill people.* (chair W.D. Boyd) London: RCP

Sainsbury Centre for Mental Health (1997) *Pulling together: the future roles and training of mental health staff.* London: Sainsbury Centre for Mental Health

Sainsbury Centre for Mental Health (1998) *Acute problems: a survey of the quality of care in acute psychiatric wards.* London: The Sainsbury Centre for Mental Health

Sainsbury Centre for Mental Health (2000) *An executive briefing on the implications of the Human Rights Act 1998 for mental health services.* London: SC for MH

United Kingdom Central Council for Nursing, Midwifery and Health Visiting (1998) *Guidelines for mental health and learning disabilities nursing.* London: UKCC

Ward, M. et al (2000) *The nursing, midwifery and health visiting contribution to the continuing care of people with mental health problems.* London: United Kingdom Central Council for Nursing, Midwifery and Health Visiting

9 Disabilities

Department of Health (1991) *Caring for people: community care in the next decade and beyond - mental handicap nursing.* (chair C. Cullen) London: HMSO

Summary: recommendations of the nursing profession for mental handicap services in relation to community care policy, concentrating on skills and qualifications, and cooperation with the rest of the health care team in providing services. Specific recommendations made to the Department of Health and the statutory bodies concerning development of services and education and training of staff, and collaboration with social services and the independent sector.

Further reading:
Allen, M.(1991) Cullen in a clear vision for the future...mentally handicapped nursing. *Nursing (London)* 4(29) 3

Crawford, M. (1991) New report recognises value of mental handicap nurses...Cullen report. *Nursing (London)* 4(29) 4-5

Department of Health (1995) *Health of the nation: a strategy for people with learning disabilities.* London: HMSO

Summary: this booklet is aimed at health commissioners. The first section looks at improving general health, carers, and cooperation between different service providers. Subsequent three sections examine health promotion, health surveillance and health care. Finally there are sections on the five key target areas of the Health of the Nation - heart disease, cancer, HIV and sexual health, accidents, mental illness - and their implementation in the specific context of learning disabilities services.

Disability Discrimination Act 1995: chapter 50. London: HMSO

Summary: this makes it unlawful to discriminate against disabled people in employment, goods and services, premises and accommodation, education, and transport, providing mechanisms for complaint and penalties for non-compliance.

- employment: this includes applications for work, conditions and terms of employment, employers' obligation to provide for the needs of disabled employees (with exemption for small businesses)
- goods and services: these include public places, hotels, information services, banking and insurance services and professional and trade services
- premises and accommodation: this includes providing equal access to living accommodation and work premises
- education: looks and both further and higher education and includes amendments to the *Education Act 1993* and the *Further and Higher Education Act 1992* this looks at adjustments to vehicles with detailed points on taxis, public service vehicles and rail services

The Act also provides for the establishment of a National Disability Council whose role is to advise the Secretary of State, issue codes of practice, gather information and give advice. The Act came into force in 1997

Further reading:

Bartram, M. (1997) Sign up to serve. *Nursing Management* 3(8) 12-13

Clements, Luke (1998) Acts of weakness. *Community Care* 8.1.1998 26-7

Memel, David and Francis, Kate (2000) The Disability Discrimination Act: an opportunity more than threat. *British Journal of General Practice* 50(461) 950-51

Stanton, B. (1997) The Disability Discrimination Act in practice. *British Journal of Health Care Management* 3(2) 106-8

Mental Health Foundation (1996) *Building expectations: opportunities and services for people with a learning disability.* London: Mental Health Foundation

Summary: many learning disabled people live in the community, but do not always get the recognition of their needs and their potential to contribute to society. This report encourages that recognition and makes recommendations about services and opportunities. Key aspects of the report include recommending new government funding for both services and staff training, and cooperation between health and social services. Other areas which are given attention include independent living, training and employment, recreation activities, and advocacy. The appointment of care managers and keyworkers to assess the needs of those with learning disabilities in all these areas, and to arrange services, is strongly recommended.

Further reading:

Leifer, D. (1996) Take time to explain. *Nursing Standard* 11(2) 14

McMillan, I. (1996) Special needs cry out for special care. *Nursing Times* 92(39) 19

Richardson, A. (1996) A fitting response. *Health Service Journal* 106(5527) 29

NHS Executive (1998) *Signposts for success in commissioning and providing health services for people with learning disabilities.* London: Department of Health

Summary: describes the role of the NHS and local authority social services in the provision of learning disability services, both now and in their future roles. The document provides guidelines for health service commissioners and providers and gives recommendations for good practice in specific areas such as children, and also epilepsy and other physical disabilities. The end of the document contains eleven pages of further reading and addresses of useful organisations.

Further reading:

Parrish, A. (1998) Exploring the NHS executive document 'Signposts for success'. *British Journal of Nursing* 7(8) 478-80

Thomas, D. (1998) Signposting the way forward. *Mental Health Care* 1(7) 224

Department of Health (1999) *Facing the facts: services for people with learning difficulties: a policy impact study of social care and health studies.* London: The Stationery Office

Summary: this report is the result of a survey carried out in 1998/9 in twenty four local authorities and partner health authorities. Findings are that progress has been made since 1992 when guidance on people with learning difficulties was issued to health and social services. They include observations on overall vision and change, accommodation and care, employment and day services, health services, protection from abuse, commissioning of services, expenditure, care management and performance management. However a considerable amount still needs to be done: between the authorities service is inconsistent and of variable quality. The report concludes that whilst examples of good practice can be found in most areas, these are usually on a small scale and national objectives and achievement targets are needed.

Disability Rights Commission Act 1999: chapter 17. London: The Stationery Office

Summary: this arose from a consultation paper: *Promoting disabled people's rights (1998).* The Act provides for a Disability Rights Commission with the following powers:

- to work on the elimination of discrimination against disabled people
- to promote equal opportunities
- improve the treatment of disabled people
- to review the *Disability Discrimination Act 1995*
- to undertake formal investigations
- offer advice and support to disabled people, employers and service providers
- promote the rights of disabled people

Further reading:
Department of Health (1998) *Promoting disabled people's rights: creating a Disability Rights Commission fit for the C21st (cm3977).* London: The Stationery Office

Jackson, C. (2000) Right on our side. *Mental Health and Learning Disabilities Care* 4(1) 6-8

Revans, L. (2000) Commission seeks to add to its remit. *Community Care* 14.9.2000 12

Carers and Disabled Children Act 2000: chapter 16. London: The Stationery Office

Summary: provides for local authorities to supply services direct to carer even when the person cared for has refused assessment or help; local authorities to have the power to make payments direct to carers even those aged 16-17, to pay those in the role of parent to disabled children and to 16-17 year old disabled young people. Following a needs assessment, carers may receive direct payments to cover costs of services, including education. The Act provides for a short term break voucher scheme as a way of lending flexibility to planning respite care.

Further reading:
Howard, M. (2001) *Paying the price: carers, poverty and social exclusion.* London: Child Poverty Action Group

Department of Health (2001) *Valuing people: a new strategy for learning disabilities for the 21st century (cm5086).* London: Department of Health

Summary: the first white paper to be published in learning disabilities for thirty years. The paper takes a broad approach, looking at people from childhood to old age, with proposals involving every government agency: housing, health and social care, education etc. Current problems boil down to issues of social exclusion, inconsistency in provision of services that are unresponsive to need, poor management, insufficient qualified staff and inadequate connexions between the various agencies.

The ten proposals are based on four principles:

- civil rights
- independence
- choice
- inclusion

The proposals include:

- an integrated, interagency approach to services for children with disabilities
- a National Information Centre
- accommodation: choice in housing and accommodation in the community for those who still remain in long-term hospitals
- a Health Action Plan for every disabled person
- a programme to modernise day services
- to increase employment opportunities
- person-centred planning: a new approach to planning care and services for individuals
- local councils to take lead responsibility in coordinating local services

Further reading:

Burns, J. (2001) Welcome to the 21st century. *Open Mind* Nov/Dec 2001 12-3

Community Living (2001) 14(4 supplement) whole issue

Gates, B. (2001) Valuing people: long awaited strategy for people with learning disabilities for the 21st century in England. *Journal of Learning Disabilities* 5(3) 203-7

Hendey, N. and Pascall, G. for the Joseph Rowntree Foundation (2002) *Disability and the transition to adulthood: achieving independent living.* Brighton: Pavilion

Summary: findings from a study of 72 young adults with disability:

- getting work, running a home, citizenship and having a social life is very difficult
- combining any two of the above especially difficult
- those who succeed usually dependent on parents and family for success
- social housing is rarely feasible because of the cost
- support for gaining and staying in employment very patchy, work environments very difficult
- some could work with personal assistance but the cost is usually prohibitive
- once found, employment was very rewarding

Clark, J. (2003) *Independence matters: an overview of the performance of social care services for physically and sensory disabled people.* London: Department of Health Social Services Inspectorate

Summary: based on information gathered in year 2002-3, the social model of disability states that social and environmental barriers limit and interfere with disabled people's need to play an integral part in society on an equal basis with others. The report takes four themes: independence at home, identity and belonging, active citizenship, systems and processes. Areas for improvement include:

- home care is often inflexible and unreliable and doesn't promote independence
- waiting times for equipment and adaptations are far too long
- services for brain-injured people are poorly developed
- there is poor support for disabled parents
- day services need to be inclusive and linked to employment opportunities
- not enough people are receiving direct payments

Audit Commission (2003) *Services for disabled children: a review of services for disabled children and their families.* London: Audit Commission

Summary: the review found that children want to be listened to and respected; they hate being excluded from ordinary activity and want the freedom to play, have friends and be safe and comfortable. Their parents have 'practical, realistic' ideas about how their and their children's experience might improve but services are found to be inconsistent and variable geographically, too often responding only to those who 'shout the loudest'. Parents report long waits for information services, equipment services are uncoordinated and confusing. In some areas there is excellent, innovative care. Recommendations include:

- services should be needs-led and focused on participating in everyday life
- there should be recognition of the special burden on children having to wait for everything
- there should be partnership working
- real progress takes leadership, better management and an attitude that is intolerant of exclusion

Further reading:
Audit Commission (2003) *Let me be me: a handbook for managers and staff working with disabled children and their families.* London: Audit Commission

Supplementary Reading

Association of Directors of Social Services et al (2002) *Deaf children: positive practice standards in social services.* London: National Deaf Children's Society and Royal National Institute for Deaf People

Cox, C. and Pearson, M. (1995) *Made to care: the case for residential and village communities for people with a mental handicap.* London: The Rannoch Trust

Department of Health (1995) *Learning disability: meeting needs through targeting skills.* London: HMSO

Emerson, E. (1994) *Moving out: the impact of relocation from hospital to community on the quality of life of people with learning disabilities.* London: HMSO

Emerson, E. et al (1996) *Residential provision for people with learning disabilities: summary report.* Manchester: University of Manchester

Jones, S. et al (2002) *Making it work: strategies for success in supported employment for people with learning difficulties.* London: Joseph Rowntree Foundation

Kay, B. Rose, S. and Turnbull, J. (1995) *Continuing the commitment: the report of the Learning Disability Nursing Project.* London: HMSO

Kay, B. et al (1996) *Learning disability nursing project resource package.* London: HMSO

McIntosh, B. (ed)(1998) *Days of change: a practical guide to developing better day opportunities with people with learning difficulties.* London: King's Fund

McIntosh, B and Whittaker, A. (2000) *Unlocking the future: developing new lifestyles with people who have complex disabilities.* London: King's Fund

Services for people with learning disabilities and challenging behaviour or mental health problems: report of a project group (1993). (chair J. L. Mansell) London: HMSO

UKCC (1998) *Guidelines for mental health and learning disability nursing.* London: UKCC

Wertheimer, A. (1996) *Changing days: developing new daytime opportunities for people who have learning difficulties.* London: King's Fund

10 Education

The National Committee of Inquiry into Higher Education (1997) *Higher education in the learning society.* (chair Ron Dearing) London: HMSO

Summary: the last Conservative government appointed this committee in 1996 to report on long-term developments, including funding arrangements, for higher education in the next twenty years. The proposal that undergraduate students contribute £1,000 towards tuition costs only affected nursing and midwifery students on degree programmes, not diploma students who continued to be funded by bursaries. To encourage prospective candidates to these programmes, the Labour government subsequently stated that degree students would also be eligible for bursaries. The report touches on many other areas of significance to education in the health professions, and recommendations are made that extend to all of higher education, some already in place in nursing and midwifery education. Recommendations include:

- encouraging research and increasing the funding to support this
- all university lecturers to have a teaching qualification
- encouraging lifelong learning
- widening access gates so as to encourage those with evidence of appropriate experience even where they have no formal qualifications. This ties in with AP(E)L initiatives and stresses the value of vocational experience and "learning from life"
- encouraging equality of access, including students with disabilities and from minority groups
- widening credit transfer between institutions and disciplines
- encouraging the use of portfolios
- regular assessment by the Quality Assurance Agency to maintain academic standards

Further reading:

Castledine, G. (1997) Impact of Dearing on the future of nurse education. *British Journal of Nursing* 6(17) 1016

Viccars, A. (1997) Midwifery education: how will the changes in funding affect both the student midwife and the midwifery lecturer? *MIDIRS Midwifery Digest* 7(4) 27-31

Whittle, T. and C. (1997) Get in the right lane. *Nursing Standard* 12(8) 24-5

Council of Deans and Heads of UK Faculties for Nursing, Midwifery and Health Visiting (1998) *Breaking the boundaries: educating nurses, midwives and health visitors for the next millennium: a position paper.* London: Council of Deans and Heads of UK Faculties for Nursing, Midwifery and Health Visiting

Summary: a radical look at the future education of nurses, midwives and health visitors working towards an all-graduate profession that is complemented by a rewarding and clearly structured clinical career. The paper recognises that there are recruitment and retention problems and is concerned about the number of students who complete courses but choose not to register to practice. Skilled individuals should be employed to develop a more regionally driven workforce plan for England. Other points include:

- regulation, supervision and education of health care assistants are inadequate and should be statutory
- life-long learning should be encouraged
- in the main, nurses and midwives are trained to work in hospitals although government policy puts the focus on primary health care
- there are problems of contracting for education where staff are developing clinical academic careers and research
- the Council supports the proposal for a single regulatory body responsible for the protection of the public, self-regulation, standard-setting, and the implementation and regulation of professional conduct
- the Council supports the establishment of an Academy of Faculties to agree standards of advanced practice
- the Council supports a central initiative to evaluate and promote interprofessional education and shared learning

Warner, Morton et al (1999) *Healthcare futures 2010: report commissioned by the UKCC Education Commission.* Glamorgan: Welsh Institute for Health and Social Care

Summary: a look at the issues of health care in the next 10 years in order to prepare pre-registration nursing and midwifery education for the future.

- Part A looks at the key elements of future health care such as: demographic changes, the changing nature of the workforce and technology.
- Part B looks at what are likely to be certain changes as opposed to guesses.
- Part C describes 3 scenarios of possible future health care: 1) 'muddling through' - making the best of things in spite of constraints on expenditure and pressure for efficiency 2) 'economic strength and consumer choice' - high expenditure with greater consumer empowerment and decision-making and 3) 'individual choice and the free market' - the NHS reduced to the safety net of a fundamentally private service.
- Part D offers a series of paradoxes: determinants of the future that may co-exist. These include: emphasis on prevention yet great demand for cure and palliation; demand for high-tech medicine yet demand for complementary therapy, greater incidence of the diseases of old age yet greater demands from younger people. Key issues will definitely include: more older people and diseases of old age, developments in genetics, increase in evidence-based practice, new ways of transferring information, changing roles and expectations in the workforce.

Within education: the common core of competencies should now include an understanding of: epidemiology, genetics, change management and information technology, and nurses and midwives will need to be trained to analyse and synthesise such scientific knowledge as a basis of decision-making.

UKCC (1999) *Fitness for practice: the UKCC commission for nursing and midwifery education.*(chair Leonard Peach) London: UKCC

Summary: the commission was established in 1998 to propose a 'way forward for pre-registration education that enabled fitness for practice based on health care need'. The principles of Project 2000 remain sound and should continue to underpin pre-registration education but the commission has reservations about recruitment and selection, the gap between theory and practice, practice placements, evaluation of outcomes and joint working between service and education. Recommendations:

- increasing flexibility in recruitment so as to attract students of different vocational and academic backgrounds; also increasing the number of graduate places but without turning nursing into an all-graduate profession
- APEL to map academic and practice credits: students who have successfully completed the first year should be able to transfer their academic and practice courses to other credit frameworks
- involving service providers in recruitment and selection
- the common foundation programme to last one year with students able to choose their branch programme either at point of recruitment or during the first year
- closing the theory practice gap by refocusing on outcomes-based competencies, these outcomes to be agreed jointly between service and education providers
- students to keep evidence-based portfolios, and to be assessed on performance in practice
- longer practice placements, reflecting the twentyfour-hour, seven-days a week working practice of the health service
- subject benchmarking in higher education to be run jointly by the QAA and UKCC to address issues specific to nursing and midwifery
- examining the possibility of skills laboratories that would prepare students for practice placements
- service and education providers to formalise support and feedback for mentors and preceptors
- students to be competent to practice at the point of registration and to have three months supervised practice at the end of their programme with full induction and preceptorship on qualification
- service and education providers to agree ownership of the responsibility for practice based education
- education purchasers to appoint an accountable individual to liaise between service and education providers and to support practice placements and contract monitoring
- developing teams of expert practitioners and academic staff to offer advice on clinical practice, management, assessment, mentoring and research

Most proposals can be implemented within two to three years. Issues such as interprofessional learning and teaching, reviewing the branch structure and funding need to be looked at on a longer term basis.

Further reading:
Anon (1999) UKCC education review supports Project 2000. *Nursing Standard* 13(52) 4-5

Munro, R. (1999) Education heads back to basics. *Nursing Times* 95(37) 5

Waters, A. (1999) A little fine tuning. *Nursing Standard* 13(52) 12-13

Department of Health (2000) *A health service of all the talents: developing the NHS workforce.* London: Department of Health

Summary: this review applies to the NHS in England only and is concerned with the roles and responsibilities of NHS staff to maximise quality of patient care, to improve training opportunities and to clarify who should be responsible for workforce planning. Some current weaknesses are identified: not enough attention given to the changing needs of the NHS; not enough flexibility about services, professional roles and training. Four key areas are identified for change:

1. Greater integration, more flexibility: workforce planning should be considered alongside local service needs for primary, secondary and tertiary care. Funding for the education of the different professions should no longer be separate. There should be greater emphasis on skill mix and healthcare worker roles.

2. Better management: local trusts should still develop their own workforce plans; in addition health authorities should contribute to the aims of the Health Improvement Programmes. New Workforce Development Confederations should be established to align the needs of local plans and non-NHS workforce needs, and to liaise with educational institutions.

3. Improved training, education and regulation: there should be flexible, multi-disciplinary training routes and programmes for all health professionals. The recommendations of *Making a difference (1999)* to be implemented. Private sector employers should also play a role in training.

4. Staff numbers and career pathways: the workforce has been underestimated and needs to increase and there should be a review of the roles of senior house officers, specialist registrars, consultants and the primary care professions.

These proposals are intended to improve patient care by the inception of true multi-disciplinary working and the end of 'professional tribes'.

Further reading:
Carlisle, D. (2000) Workforce plans see managers in control. *Health Service Journal* 110 (5700) 7

Committee of Vice Chancellors and Principals (2000) *CVCP response to the consultation on 'A health service of all the talents'.* London: CVCP

Glen, S. (2000) Partnerships: the way forward. *Nurse Education Today* 20(5) 339-40

Audit Commission (2001) *Hidden talents: education, training and development for healthcare staff in NHS trusts. London: Audit Commission*

Summary: this covers the education and training of all existing healthcare staff in NHS trusts except dentists and doctors - see *The doctors' tale (1995)*. A partner study conducted by the National Audit Office looks at the provision of education for newly qualified healthcare professionals. Education and training is commonly provided 'in-house' and by commission through higher education institutions. It covers core and advanced specialist skills as well as common skills to do with information handling and technology, management and interpersonal skills. There is a need for consistent education and training because of:

- the national shortage of nurses and other health care professionals in the NHS
- the need to prepare existing staff at all levels to cope with the changes brought about by modernisation
- changes in professional regulation

Twenty three recommendations are aimed at all levels of personnel from individuals to senior management and are designed to promote a commitment to lifelong learning. They are based on the following principles:

- identifying needs
- facilitating education and training
- monitoring, reviewing and evaluating

Further reading:
Munro, R. (2001) Your career development still decided by a postcode lottery. *Nursing Times* 97(9) 10-12

National Audit Office (2001) *Educating and training the future health professional workforce for England.* London: National Audit Office

Summary: where the Audit Commission's report looks at provision for existing NHS staff, this report looks at education and training for new staff - pre-registration. The *NHS plan (2000)* notes that staff shortages are the biggest restraint on the development of the NHS whilst *A health service of all the talents (2000)* shows how underestimates in workforce development and planning have led to these shortages. There are also found to be variations across the country in the cost per student of qualifying and whilst the 20% attrition rates are no worse in health care than any other higher education subject, this represents a waste of resources and the Department of Health has therefore set a target of 13% attrition or less. The report offers recommendations to the Department of Health, the NHS, higher education institutions and the Workforce Development Confederations. These come under the headings of:

- better planning and commissioning of education and training
- obtaining value for money
- developing effective inter-agency partnerships

Department of Health (2001) *Working together, learning together: a framework for lifelong learning in the NHS.* London: Department of Health

Summary: taking as its basis the principle that lifelong learning enables staff growth and fulfilment, organisational effectiveness and improvements in patient care, part of the brief of *The NHS plan (2000)* was to modernise education, training and development. Eight chapters cover:

1. core skills
2. the NHS as a learning organisation

3. the provision of opportunities for staff without professional qualifications

4. pre-registration education for all health care professionals: includes joint learning for core skills, flexible entry and exit points, and partnerships between health, education and regulatory bodies

5. post-registration and professional development emphasising consistent standards and work-based learning

6. effective leadership and management

7. everything an organisation needs to promote lifelong learning: mentorship, supervision, investment and electronic delivery: here outlining the role of the proposed NHS University that will offer '24/365' access to learning opportunities

8. a five year plan of action

Further reading:
Robinson, S. and Murrells, T. (2002) What do newly qualified staff think of preceptorship? *Employing Nurses and Midwives* May 2002 13-4

Department for Education and Skills (2003) *The future of higher education (cm5735).* London: The Stationery Office

Summary: in the face of pressure to succeed and a growing challenge from other countries, higher education (HE) faces the following issues:

*   HE must adapt to the need for new skills

*   the class gap at university is still wide

*   compared with our competitors HE is under funded: between 1989 and 1997 funding per student dropped 36%

*   HE needs stronger links with business

*   HE institutions struggle to employ the best minds and academics

*   there is an estimated £8 billion backlog in teaching and research facilities

Plans for reform include:

*   increase spending on research and reward research work, creating an Arts and Humanities Research Council

*   support and invest in the relationship with the business world

*   reward and support high quality teaching, using student choice to drive quality and establishing a Teaching Quality Academy to set new national professional standards

*   develop new kinds of qualifications such as two-year work-focused 'foundation degrees' bringing a flexible approach to support those on part-time courses

*   closing the social class gap: grants for lower income students; universities to produce Access Agreements to benefit disadvantaged students before they raise fees; improve the AimHigher programme to strengthen HE links with schools and colleges

*   funding: from 2004 the Government will offer grants for up to £1,000 for lower income students and will continue to pay up to the first £1,100 of their fees. From 2006 a Graduate Contribution Scheme will allow universities to ask for up to £3,000 from graduates for each course. The Government will end all 'up front' payment of

tuition fees and arrange for students to repay their loans through the tax system, linked to their ability to pay. From 2005 the Government will raise from £10,000 to £15,000 the threshold at which graduates must start repaying loans. Universities will also be supported to build up their own endowment funds

Further reading:
Langlands, A. (2003) *Synchronising higher education and the NHS*. London: The Stationery Office

Higher Education Act 2004: chapter 8. London: The Stationery Office

Summary: designed to support the white paper *The future of higher education (2003)* the Act provides for:

* establishment of an Arts and Humanities Research Council replacing the existing Arts and Humanities Research Board

* a scheme to manage student complaints

* higher education institutions to set their own fees up to a set amount with the right to appeal to OFFA if they want them to be higher

* the appointment of a Director of Fair Access to Higher Education in an office know informally as Office for Fair Access (OFFA)

* preventing a student loan becoming part of their estate in a bankruptcy case

* a measure to support deferring pay-back of tuition fees - reimbursing the university up front so that students can pay later

* allowing exchange of information in relation to student support

Supplementary Reading

Ballard, Elaine (1997) *Information for caring: a framework for including health informatics in programmes of learning for nurses, midwives and health visitors and other clinical professions*. London: ENB

Department of Health and Universities UK (2002) *Funding learning and development for the healthcare workforce*. London: Department of Health

Department of Health (1989) *Working for patients: working paper 10: education and training*. London: HMSO

Engel, C. (2002) *Towards a European approach to an enhanced education of the health professionals in the C21st*. London: Centre for the Advancement of Interprofessional Education

English National Board for Nursing Midwifery and Health Visiting (1994) *Creating lifelong learners: partnerships for care*. London: ENB

English National Board and the Department of Health (2001) *Preparation of mentors and teachers: a new framework for guidance*. London: ENB

Gillam, S. et al (1999) *Building bridges: the future of GP education: developing partnerships with the service*. London: King's Fund

Hollingworth, Sheila (1997) *Lecturer practitioner roles in England: a report prepared for the Chief Nursing Officer/Director of Nursing*. London: NHS Executive

National Audit Office (1992) *Nursing education: implementation of project 2000 in England.* London: HMSO

Nursing and Midwifery Council (2002) *Guide for students of nursing and midwifery.* London: NMC

Nursing and Midwifery Council (2004) *PREP handbook.* London: NMC

Nursing and Midwifery Council (2002) *Preparation of mentors and teachers.* London: NMC

Nursing and Midwifery Council (2001) *Standards for specialist education and practice.* London: NMC

Nursing and Midwifery Council (2000) *Standards for the preparation of teachers of nursing, midwifery and specialist community public health nurses.* London: NMC

Nursing and Midwifery Council (2002) *Supporting nurses and midwives through lifelong learning.* London: NMC

Royal College of Nursing et al (1998) *Tomorrow's nurses and midwives: charter for nursing and midwifery education.* London: Royal College of Nursing

UKCC (1994) *The future of professional practice: the Council's standards for education March 1994.* London: UKCC

UKCC (1986) *Project 2000: a new preparation for practice.* London: UKCC

UKCC (1990) *The report of the post-registration education and practice project.* London: UKCC

11 Ethical Issues and Human Rights

Human Tissue Act 1961: chapter 54. London: HMSO

Summary: allows the use of all or parts of a body for therapeutic, research or educational purposes provided consent has been given orally or in writing by the dying person in front of two witnesses. After death the same may occur if after making "reasonable" enquiries, whoever possesses the body is convinced the patient or their spouse had no objection. The Act also regulates post mortem examinations.

Abortion Act 1967: chapter 87. London: HMSO

Summary: the *Offences Against the Person Act 1861* made abortion a criminal offence even for medical reasons. Offences were punishable by imprisonment for between three years and life, for mother or doctor. the *Infant Life Preservation Act 1929* allowed a termination if it was to preserve the life of the mother, unless the foetus was capable of being born live which was seen as from 28 weeks in which case it was illegal. The 1967 Act permits termination in the following circumstances:

1. if continuing with a pregnancy presents greater risk to a mother than abortion
2. if it is to prevent serious injury to the physical or mental health of the mother
3. if continuation of pregnancy holds greater risk of injury to the physical or mental health of the woman than would a termination
4. if continuing with the pregnancy involves risk to the mental or physical health of any existing children
5. if there is serious risk the child would be born with physical or mental abnormalities or in emergency, if it is deemed necessary by operating practitioners
6. if it is to save the life of the woman
7. if it is to prevent serious permanent injury to the pregnant woman

The *Human Fertilisation and Embryology Act 1990* (see below) brought a limit of 24 weeks to circumstances 3 and 4. The circumstances in 1, 2 and 5 are without time limit.

Further reading:

Dimond, B. (1999) A legal right to abortion: right or wrong? *British Journal of Midwifery* 7(6) 355-7

Moore, A. (1997) A change that is here to stay: the impact of the abortion law over the last 30 years. *Nursing Standard* 12(6) 22-3

Moore, A. (1997) Gin and despair: working life of doctors and nurses before the 1967 Abortion Act. *Health Service Journal* 107(5567) 28-9

Sex Discrimination Act 1975: chapter 65. London: The Stationery Office

Summary: with a few exceptions, the Act prohibits discrimination against men and women of any age (including children), on the grounds of gender. It also prohibits discrimination against people who are married, but not against people who are not married. If someone exercises their rights under the Act, victimisation is prohibited. The Act applies to discrimination in employment, education, goods, services and premises and it provides for the establishment of an Equal Opportunities Commission.

Race Relations Act 1976: chapter 74. London: The Stationery Office

Summary: with very few exceptions the Act makes it unlawful to discriminate against anyone on the grounds of race, colour, nationality, ethnic or national origin and outlaws segregation, victimisation and harassment on the same grounds. It applies to discrimination in employment, education, housing and the provision of good and services. It imposes a duty on all public bodies to promote equal opportunities and good relations and provides for a Commission for Racial Equality.

Anatomy Act 1984: chapter 14. London: HMSO

Summary: allows a person to bequeath their body for use in an educational setting. Bodies may be dissected and examined, but not used to practice surgical technique. Such bodies must be disposed of within three years according to the donor's wishes (buried or cremated). The Act also provides for an HM Inspector of Anatomy to oversee these activities, inspect premises and check on disposal practices.

Human Organs Transplant Act 1989: chapter 31. London: HMSO

Summary: makes it a criminal offence to have commercial dealings in organs for transplant and an offence to advertise the buying and selling of organs. The Act also prohibits the removal of an organ from a living person for transplant unless they the donor are genetically related to the receiver. Published in the same year, the Human Organs Transplants (unrelated persons) Regulations 1989, allows donations between non-blood relatives (e.g. husband and wife) at the approval of ULTRA: the Unrelated Live Transplant Regulatory Authority.

Human Fertilisation and Embryology Act 1990: chapter 37. London: The Stationery Office

Summary: provides for the licensing and monitoring of fertility treatment that involves the use of donated sperm, eggs or embryos created outside the body (i.e. in vitro). It provides for time-limited storage of sperm, eggs and embryos; and for regulating research on embryos, the purpose of which must be confined to knowledge about the causes of miscarriage, congenital diseases, detection of abnormalities and the advancement of infertility treatments. It also licenses centres for preimplanted genetic diagnosis. The Act provides for the creation of the Human Fertilisation and Embryology Authority to oversee all related activities and to review developments in the field. It defines the rights of donors, mothers, and children, whose rights are paramount.

Further reading:
McLean, S. (1997) *Consent and the law: review of the current provisions in the Human Fertilisation and Embryology Act 1990 for the UK Health Ministers.* Glasgow: University of Glasgow

Human Fertilisation and Embryology (Disclosure of Information) Act 1992: chapter 54. London: HMSO

Summary: the purpose of the Act is to relax the confidentiality provisions set in the original *Human Fertilisation and Embryology Act 1990* (see above). Passing information from licensed centres without consent is prohibited. Disclosure should usually only involve one person (e.g. a GP) and usually only in connexion with providing treatment or medical services, or to prevent imminent danger to that person.

Stillbirth (Definition) Act 1992: chapter 29. London: HMSO

Summary: reduces the gestational age when a baby is recognised as stillborn from 28 to 24 weeks. Previously, terminations of pregnancy between 24 and 28 weeks, were treated as miscarriages for statistical purposes and are now considered stillbirths.

Public Interest Disclosure Act 1998: chapter 23. London: The Stationery Office

Summary: this came into force in 1999 as an addition to the *Employment Rights Act 1996.* The Act is designed to protect from victimisation individuals who speak out (or 'whistleblow') in the interests of public safety. Provisions include:

- the meanings and circumstances surrounding disclosure, for instance disclosure does not qualify if it involves an individual breaking the law or if it is made purely for personal gain
- employees may bring a complaint to an Employment Tribunal and be compensated for unfair dismissal, redundancy or any other kind of victimisation
- 'gagging' clauses in contracts and severance agreements will be void

Health Service Circular 1999/198 outlines how the Act will apply to the NHS. All organisations are advised to write local whistleblowing policies.

Further reading:
Bradbury, J. (2003) Whistle while you work. *Nursing Management* 10(4) 13-5

Snell, J. (1998) Blowing in the wind. *Health Service Journal* 108(5619) 20-23

Taylor, H. / NHSE (1999) *The Public Interest Disclosure Act 1998: whistleblowing in the NHS.* (HSC 1999/198) Leeds: Department of Health

Vickers, L. (1999) Freedom of speech in the National Health Service. *Journal of Social Welfare and Family Law* 21(2) 121-134

Data Protection Act 1998: chapter 29. London: The Stationery Office

Summary: includes electronic, manual and recorded data about an individual who is a living person that can be named or identified. If identifiers are removed, the data is no longer personal and not therefore covered by the Act. The Act regulates obtaining, keeping, using and disclosing such information. Guiding principles are transparency and consent: individuals must be very clear why information is being collected and what for, and any individual may withdraw their consent at any time. Eight data protection principles:

1. personal data must be processed lawfully and

2. obtained for specified, lawful purposes
3. data may only be taken that is adequate and relevant to the purpose
4. data must be accurate and kept up to date and
5. not kept longer than necessary
6. data must be processed according to the rights of data subjects
7. measures must be taken against unlawful use of personal data and against loss, damage or destruction
8. personal data must not be transferred out of the European Community

Further reading:
Redsell, S. A. and Cheater, F. M. (1997) The Data Protection Act 1998: implications for health researchers. *Journal of Advanced Nursing* 35(4) 508-13

Human Rights Act 1998: chapter 42. London: The Stationery Office

Summary: this came into force in October 2000 and brings the *European Convention on Human Rights (1999)* into UK law. The articles are:

- right to life
- prohibition of torture
- prohibition of slavery and forced labour
- right to liberty and security
- right to a fair trial
- no punishment without law
- right to respect for private and family life
- freedom of thought, conscience and religion
- freedom of expression
- freedom of assembly and association
- right to marry
- prohibition of discrimination
- prohibition of abuse of rights

Protocols are later additions to the original convention. They are:

- protection of property
- right to education
- right to free elections
- abolition of the death penalty

Further reading:
British Medical Association (2000) *The medical profession and human rights: handbook for a changing agenda.* London: Zed Books

Council of Europe (1999) *European Convention on Human Rights and Property Rights.* Strasbourg: Council of Europe/Conseil de l'Europe

Dow, J. (2000) Human Rights Act 1998: implications for community care services. *Managing Community Care* 8(4) 24-32

International Council of Nurses (1999) *ICN on health and human rights.* Geneva: ICN

Sainsbury Centre for Mental Health (2000) *An executive briefing on the implications of the Human Rights Act 1998 for mental health services.* London: SC for MH

United Nations (1998) *Universal declaration of human rights.* Geneva: UN

Stone, D. (2000) The Human Rights Act 1998. *British Journal of Health Care Management* 6(11) 515-7

Wilkinson, R. and Caulfield, Helen (2000) *The Human Rights Act: a practical guide for nurses.* London: Whurr

Race Relations (Amendment) Act 2000: chapter 34. London: The Stationery Office

Summary: the 1976 Act made employers 'vicariously' liable for acts of discrimination committed by their employees at work. The Stephen Lawrence inquiry found that police officers had 'slipped through the net' because they were not employees but 'office holders'. On the recommendations of the inquiry therefore, this Act provides that all police officers shall be subject to race relations legislation and that Chief Officers of Police be made vicariously liable for discriminatory acts committed by their officers.

Further reading:
Home Office (1999) *The Stephen Lawrence inquiry (cm4262-I).* (chair William MacPherson) London: The Stationery Office

Freedom of Information Act 2000: chapter 36. London: The Stationery Office

Summary: follows a white paper *Your right to know.* The Act gives right of access to recorded information held by public authorities, including the NHS, schools, colleges, government, the police and others. It covers how an application should be made and how a public authority must offer advice and assistance, granting them permission to charge fees, setting time limits for fulfilling a request and specifying exemptions. The Act provides for the appointment of an Information Commissioner, to whom the public may apply directly. The Act extends to Public Records Offices, thus amending the *Public Records Act 1958* which provided for the appointment of a Keeper of the Offices, and facilities for viewing and copying records.

Further reading:
Cabinet Office (1997) *Your right to know: the Government's proposals for a freedom of information act (cm3818).* (chair Chancellor of the Duchy of Lancaster) London: The Stationery Office

Wilson, K. (2004) From secrecy to openness? *Health Service Manager Briefing* 10.8.2004 6-8

Bristol Royal Infirmary Inquiry (2001) *The report of the public inquiry into children's heart surgery at the Bristol Royal Infirmary 1984-1995: learning from Bristol (cm5207).* (chair Ian Kennedy) London: The Stationery Office

Summary: at £15m this is the longest, most comprehensive public inquiry ever held on practice in the NHS. It follows a General Medical Council inquiry into the performance of 3 consultants: Wisheart, Dhasmana and Roylance following allegations of malpractice made by consultant anaesthetist Stephen Bolsin in 1995, who implied that fear of losing funding had caused the unit to 'turn a blind eye'. That inquiry looked at complex heart operations on 53 children of whom 29 died and and 4 were left brain-damaged. Wisheart and Roylance were struck off, Dhasmana was sacked, and barred from operating on children for three years. This public inquiry's brief was:

- to look into the care and management of children under one year undergoing complex cardiac surgery at Bristol between the years 1984 and 1995
- to look into the adequacy of the whole service
- to look into what happened when concerns were raised and why they were not addressed

The Inquiry found circumstances and situations that are by no means unique to Bristol and therefore urged that its recommendations be considered by all service areas within the NHS. The 200 recommendations arise from the following issues:

- RESPECT and HONESTY: this refers to the importance of communicating with patients and families, keeping them informed, involving them in decisions of care and providing support in the process of giving consent
- LEADERSHIP: this looks at the roles of the Department of Health, NICE and CHI, the Council for Quality of Healthcare and at local level, the roles of trusts, their consultants, chief executives and senior managers
- COMPETENCE: at all levels of education and training there should be greater emphasis given to 'non-clinical' skills such as communication, reflective practice leadership and teamwork. As well as the regulating bodies - such as the GMC, NMC etc - a Council for the Regulation of Healthcare Professionals with statutory powers should integrate the different systems of professional regulation, promoting common curricula and shared learning
- SAFETY: there should be a national system for reporting events in safety and confidence, and systems for examining 'sentinel' events in order to learn from them. Throughout, the Inquiry abhors blaming and scapegoating in favour of open systems of working that can acknowledge mistakes will occur and can be learnt from
- STANDARDS: NICE to be responsible for coordinating everything related to standard-setting, noting that some standards should be compulsory and others set to be achieved over time. The role of the CHI needs further development as do the mechanisms for monitoring performance at local and national levels
- PUBLIC EMPOWERMENT: this refers to involving the public in commissioning and providing care services at all levels. It urges 'transparent' working practices by the professional bodies, and that Patient Councils, Patients' Forums and the PCTs' Patient and Advocacy Liaison Service provide for fully involving the wider public - not just existing patients

- CARE OF CHILDREN: this looks at communication with children and their parents; the need for child-centred facilities with specialist trained staff; greater integration of primary, acute and specialist care. The proposed National Service Framework should be published as a matter of urgency and must include mechanisms for setting and reviewing standards. The Inquiry also proposes appointing a National Director for Children's Healthcare Services with consideration given to creating a Children's Commissioner whose role would be to promote the rights of the child in all public areas. There are also specific recommendations to do with care of children with congenital heart disease

Further reading:

Department of Health (2002) *Learning from Bristol: the Department of Health's response to the report of the public inquiry into children's heart surgery at the Bristol Royal Infirmary 1984-1995 (cm5363).* London: The Stationery Office

Walshe, K. and Offen, N. (2001) A very public failure: lessons for quality improvement in healthcare organisations from the Bristol Royal Infirmary. *Quality in Health Care* 10(4) 250-56

Health Service Journal (2001) 111 (5764 and 5765) whole issues

Higgins, Joan (2001) The listening blank. *Health Service Journal* 111(5772) 22-25

Royal Liverpool Children's Inquiry, House of Commons (2001) *Royal Liverpool Children's Hospital Inquiry report: the Alder Hey report.* (chair Michael Redfern) London: The Stationery Office

Summary: the inquiry was called in 1999 when it was discovered that the Alder Hey and other children's hospitals had been harvesting and storing organs from deceased babies without their parents consent. Alder Hey also stored foetuses after terminations of pregnancy and stillbirths; other hospitals gave thymus glands taken from live children during heart surgery to a pharmaceutical company for research in exchange for funds. The discovery led to having to inform thousands of parents about what had happened. Where the organs could be retrieved, parents held 'second funerals' for their dead children. Recommendations include:

- looking at research agreements between universities and trusts
- reforming senior executive level arrangements and procedures
- reviewing audit procedures and managerial appointments
- looking at clinicians' dealings with coroners
- reforming the coroners' service, looking at education and training and procedures to do with authorising a post-mortem examination especially as regards consent
- amending the *Human Tissue Act 1961*, drawing up guidelines for informed consent in the health service

Further reading:

Dewar, S. and Boddington, P. (2004) Returning to the Alder Hey reporting and its reporting: addressing confusions and improving enquiries. *Journal of Medical Ethics* 30(5) 463-9

English, V. and Sommerville, A. (2003) Presumed consent for transplantation: a dead issue after Alder Hey? *Journal of Medical Ethics* 29(3) 147-52

Prior, S. (2002) Lessons learnt from illegal retention of human tissue. *Health Care Risk Report* 8(4) 12-13

Department of Health, Department for Education and Employment, Home Office and Chief Medical Officer (2001) *The removal, retention and use of human organs and tissue from post-mortem examination: advice from the CMO.* London: The Stationery Office

Summary: the result of public concern after Bristol and Liverpool parents discovered that their children's organs and tissue had been retained post-mortem without knowledge or consent. There are 17 recommendations including:

- revision of the law with amendments to ensure that consent is given and pathologists authorised to retain organs
- a code of practice with a standardised consent form and setting standards in good communications
- the appointment of an overseeing Commission of pathology practices
- controls on the import and export of body parts
- a new system of death certification involving an independent medical examiner to address issues raised by the Shipman inquiry
- bereavement support
- to promote the value of research
- research into less invasive forms of post-mortem examination

Further reading:
Dimond, Bridget (2001) Alder Hey and the retention and storage of body parts. *British Journal of Midwifery* 9(3) 173-6

Fox, M. and McHale, J. (2000) Regulating human body parts and products. *Health Care Analysis* 8(2) 83-201

Smith, Tom (2001) Push me, pull you. *Health Service Journal* 111(5747) 30-31

Woodcock, Sue (2001) Bodyparts and the law. *Nursing Times* 97(6) 32-34

Department of Health (2001) *Reference guide to consent for examination or treatment.* London: Department of Health

Summary: a guide for health professionals on the law surrounding valid consent which will be altered if the new *Mental Capacity Bill (2004)* becomes law. Guidance is given on: seeking consent; when consent is withdrawn or refused; gaining consent from 'adults without capacity' as well as children and young people; withdrawing and withholding life-prolonging treatment. Issues raised by the *Human Rights Act 1998* are considered along with removal of organs from persons declared dead.

Further reading:
Austin, Julie (2001) Whose life is it anyway?: or self-determination and the capacity to give consent to treatment. *Health Service Manager Briefing* 9.2.2001 no.64 6-8

Billcliff, N. McCabe, E. and Brown, K.W. (2001) Informed consent to medication in long-term psychiatric in-patients. *Psychiatric Bulletin* 25(4) 132-4

British Medical Association (2001) *Consent, rights and choices in health care for children and young people.* London: BMJ Books

Verity, C. and Nicoll, A. (2002) Consent, confidentiality and the threat to public health surveillance. *British Medical Journal* 324(7347) 1210-3

Human Reproductive Cloning Act 2001: chapter 23. London: The Stationery Office

Summary: makes it a criminal offence to place in the womb an embryo that was created other than by fertilisation. The occurrence had to be legislated for separately as it was found that such embryos were not governed by the *Human Fertilisation and Embryology Act 1990* (see above).

Chief Medical Officer (2001) *Harold Shipman's clinical practice 1974 - 1998.* (chair Richard Baker) London: The Stationery Office

Summary: this report an audit of Harold Shipman's clinical practice, not the full inquiry (see below). Looking at medical certificates of cause of death (MCCDs) issued by Shipman, cremation forms issued, the deaths of all Shipman's patients and his practice in prescribing controlled drugs, the audit is looking for patterns of death by age group, gender, place and time of day and the connexions between death and patient history. Findings:

- Harold Shipman issued 499 MCCDs whilst working in Hyde compared with a maximum of 210 issued by any of the other six local general practitioners
- there was an unusually high number deaths at home, among females over 65
- deaths occurred in the afternoon, with Shipman present, giving cause of death as heart disease, stroke or old age
- this pattern is evident from his first years of practice
- the connexion between cause of death and patient history appears tenuous
- the audit trail as to prescribing controlled drugs is unclear
- Shipman's record-keeping was poor

Recommendations include:
- the monitoring of general practitioners to be reviewed so as to include death rates, prescribing controlled drugs and record keeping
- a system is needed to gather information on numbers of deaths and MCCDs issued
- MCCDs must include a brief record of cause and circumstances of death as well as a brief patient history
- GP validation should include assessment of record-keeping
- the storage of clinical records must be reviewed
- GP's controlled drugs register should be open to inspection
- patient records and GP's and pharmacists' controlled drugs registers should note batch numbers

Further reading:

Baker, R. et al (2003) Monitoring mortality rates in general practice after Shipman. *British Medical Journal* 326(7383) 274-6

Carey, Penny (2001) Getting away with it. *Health Care Risk Report* 7(6) 20-1

Caverford, Cathy (2001) Spectre of Shipman still haunts GPs. *Doctor* 8.2.2001 40-42

Ramsay, Sarah (2001) Audit further exposes UK's worst serial killer. *The Lancet* 357(9250) 123-4

The Shipman Inquiry (2002) *First report: death disguised.* (chair Janet Smith) London The Stationery Office

Summary: between March 1975 and June 1998, Dr Harold Shipman killed 215 of his patients of whom 171 were women and 44 were men. Most were killed by a lethal dose of an opiate. Most of Shipman's victims were elderly, the youngest was a 41-year old man suffering from terminal illness and Shipman 'hastened' his death. The youngest person to die unexpectedly was 47 years old. The Inquiry investigated 888 deaths altogether, and found strong reasons to suspect 45 other deaths, but insufficient evidence to be absolutely certain.

The Shipman Inquiry (2003) *Second report: the police investigation of March 1998 (cm5853).* (chair Janet Smith) London: The Stationery Office

Summary: the report focuses on a police investigation that was initiated when a neighbouring GP raised concerns about the number of deaths coming from Shipman's practice, as well as the nature of their dying. The report finds the police involved were inexperienced and unfit for the case, failing to pursue key lines of investigation such as when two bodies were available for autopsy but not followed up. A doctor was asked to review the records of some of Shipman's patients and failed to see a pattern simply because he could not entertain the idea that Shipman was a murderer. The report highlights this 'credibility gap' as leading to unacceptable negligence overall. Had the investigation proceeded as it should, three lives may have been saved.

The Shipman Inquiry (2003) *Third report: death certification and the investigation of deaths by coroners (cm5854).* (chair Janet Smith) London: The Stationery Office

Summary: looks at our system for registering deaths and certifying cremation and at the way coroners investigate deaths. In the context of the Shipman inquiry the report finds loopholes at every stage, preventing the detection of error, malpractice or neglect. Recommendations include:

- a nationally agreed policy for handling death in the community, managed by the Coroner's office, covering the roles of ambulance, police and medical staff
- death certification needs regulation: 'death by natural causes' is not an acceptable statement; clarity is needed about when to report a death
- coroners should cross-check cause of death on certificates with person other than the certifying doctor

- coroners are usually either medics or lawyers but they need training for expertise in both areas before they come into post. They also need the support of a team of trained investigating officers
- inquests should only be in public where there is a public health concern, a coroner's report should be enough otherwise
- other recommendations concern the procedures for registering death, cremation certification and autopsy

Further reading:

Baker, R. (2004) Patient-centred care after Shipman. *Journal of the Royal Society of Medicine* 97(4) 161-5

Berry, C. (2003) Death certification and Dr Shipman. *Medicine Science and the Law* 43(3) 193-4

Houghton, G. (2004) 'Last seen before death': the unrecognised clue in the Shipman case. *Quality in Primary Care* 12(1) 5-11

Review of Coroner Services (2003) *Death certification and investigation in England and Wales and Northern Ireland: the report of a fundamental review 2003 (cm5831).* (chair Tom Luce) London: The Stationery Office

Young, J.G. (2004) Speaking for the dead to protect the living: the roles of the coroner and the Shipman inquiry. *British Journal of General Practice* 54(500) 162-3

The Shipman Inquiry (2004) *Fourth report: the regulation of controlled drugs in the community (cm6249).* (chair Janet Smith) London: The Stationery Office

Summary: gives an account of Shipman's pethidine addiction in the 1970's when he regularly prescribed pethidine for patients but kept the drugs for himself. In 1976 he was found guilty of eight counts of unlawful possession of a schedule two drug (he asked for 74 other offences to be taken into account) but in spite of this he was not monitored or restricted from keeping and prescribing controlled drugs when he returned to practice in 1977. The majority of Shipman's victims were killed by lethal doses of diamorphine. Shipman was regularly dispensed 30mg ampoules of diamorphine, a dose that is too strong for treating acute pain and too weak for the chronic pain of terminal illness. He regularly stole and stored diamorphine by prescribing it for 'cancer patients' who were either already dead or did not need the drug. Recommendations include:

- establishing a controlled drugs inspectorate to monitor and audit how doctors and pharmacists prescribe and store controlled drugs
- regulate the prescribing rights of GPs, the use of prescription forms and record keeping
- it should be a criminal offence to self-prescribe a schedule 2 drug

Further reading:

Anon (2004) Shipman inquiry criticisms that could sink the GMC. *Pulse* 64(9) 16-7

Bellingham, C. (2003) Shipman inquiry: views on tightening of controlled drug regulations sought. *Pharmaceutical Journal* 271(7261) 171-2

Department of Health and Home Office (2004) *Safer management of controlled drugs: the Government response to the 4th report of the Shipman inquiry.* London: Department of Health

The Shipman Inquiry (2004) *The fifth report: safeguarding patients: lessons from the past – proposals for the future (cm6394).* (chair Janet Smith) London: The Stationery Office

Summary: the 1300-page report looked at the responsibilities of primary care organisations and the General Medical Council in relation to Shipman's crimes. Although neither are seen as directly responsible, the report is highly critical of the GMC whose 'flawed' practices are seen as 'looking after their own': acting in the interests of doctors rather than focussing on the protection of patients. 100 recommendations look at:

- handling complaints and managing disciplinary procedures
- using prescribing information, mortality and the investigation of complaints as clinical governance measures
- recruiting and appointing GPs and making their personal files available to the NHS, the Department of Health and the GMC
- supporting small and single-doctor practices

Specific recommendations include:

- an independent selection process for medical and lay members of the GMC
- doctors' 'fitness to practice' to be reviewed on a regular basis as part of re-registering
- the creation of a database about every working doctor including details of any disciplinary action
- patients should be able to find out about a doctor's registration and their fitness to practice
- patients should have the right to refuse to be treated by a doctor who has been struck or suspended from the register in the past

In the light if the Shipman and other inquiries, the GMC began a process of reform in 2003, aiming for greater accountability and transparency. However, the report is sceptical that this will be enough to make a significant difference. Six doctors who signed Shipman's cremation forms face disciplinary action for misconduct. The Government is expected to respond to the report early in 2005.

Female Genital Mutilation Act 2003: chapter 31. London: The Stationery Office

Summary: this Act replaces the *Prohibition of Female Circumcision Act 1985* and makes it an offence to mutilate a woman's/girl's external genitals unless it be by an approved person directly for her well-being, or as an unavoidable part of surgery performed when she is in labour or has given birth. In determining her wellbeing a person may not take into account her or someone else's belief that such an operation is necessary. The Act makes it an offence to aid or abet any woman to perform such mutilation herself. It is unlawful for a UK national to perform such surgery abroad, as is a non-UK person performing the operation on a UK woman or girl overseas. Penalties for offences include imprisonment for up to 14 years.

Further reading:

Hellsten, S.K. (2004) Rationalising circumcision: from tradition to fashion, from public health to individual freedom: critical notes on the cultural persistence of the practice of genital mutilation. *Journal of Medical Ethics* 30(3) 248-53

Department of Health (2003) *Human bodies, human choices: summary of responses to the consultation report.* London: Department of Health

Summary: the consultation looked at issues of consent; the use of human material for education and research; compliance and the penalties for non-compliance; special issues such as the use of cell lines and stem cells, foetal tissue and organ transplantation from dead and living persons.

- consent: should be at the basis of any legislation on the principle of gift - i.e. not commerce - and there should be specific consent made for material used for research
- as long as consent is given, it must be possible to use human material for education, research and training
- transplants: there should be a single system applying to living or dead donors, with donation seen as an unconditional gift, making it illegal to sell or advertise organs
- there should be one system of supervision conducted by one authority, with penalties for non-compliance including prison sentences
- it should not be possible to profit financially from tissue donation
- it should be possible to save the gametes of a child or adult for their own future use but not someone else's
- the wishes of the donor should prevail
- there should be public education to promote understanding of the need and usefulness of post mortem examination, and there should be research into less invasive post mortem methods

Further reading:

Department of Health (2002) *Human bodies, human choices: the law on human organs in England and Wales: a consultation report.* London: Department of Health

Department of Health (2003) *Investigation of events that followed the death of Cyril Mark Isaacs.* London: The Stationery Office

Department of Health (2003) *Saving lives, valuing donors: a transplant framework for England.* London: Department of Health

Department of Health (2003) *Our inheritance, our future: realising the potential of genetics in the NHS (cm579 - I & II).* London: The Stationery Office

Summary: a greater understanding of genetics has lead to more accurate diagnosis, tailored prediction of predisposition to illnesses; new therapies, and the ability to focus treatments according to a person's genetic profile. Because of genetic variation, individuals respond differently to drugs and in the field of pharmacogenetics, in the next five years patients could be tested for this response in order that any prescribed medicine is 'right first time'. In the next five-to-ten years, gene therapy will involve the deliberate introduction of genetic material to treat diseases. In order that the NHS keeps abreast of developments, the paper sets out a three year plan looking at:

- strengthening specialist services, increasing investment and capacity of laboratory and genetics services

- integrating genetics into everyday practice: introducing genetics centres for genetics clinicians, counsellors and laboratories

- promote understanding and reassure the public through openness in policy-making

- support research, investing in pharmacogenetics and gene therapies

Further reading:
Royal College of Midwives (2003) *Response to the Government white paper 'Our inheritance, our future: realising the potential of genetics in the NHS.* London: RCM

Human Fertilisation and Embryology (Deceased Fathers) Act 2003: chapter 24. London: The Stationery Office

Summary: allows for the acknowledgement of a father in the event of a child being conceived and born after his death and as the result of using his sperm or using a stored embryo created with his sperm before he died. It does not apply to a situation where a man dies during a normal pregnancy. The Act was instigated so that a child born in these circumstances would not have any rights (such as nationality or inheritance) that might impede winding up the deceased man's estate. Under the Act any man wanting to be recorded as the father of a child, born in this way after his death, must give written consent to the use of his sperm and to being treated as the father. The mother must also write and sign a declaration within 42 days of the birth that she wishes the man to be recorded as the child's father.

House of Lords (2003) *Patients' Protection Bill.* London: The Stationery Office

Summary: offering food and drink (sustenance) is seen as part of performing a duty of care for anyone looking after a patient. The Bill would prevent anyone responsible for a patient either withdrawing or withholding sustenance with the intention of hastening their death. It would not be treated as an offence if the patient requested that sustenance be withdrawn or if he refused sustenance. Likewise in the case of a patient incapable of consenting, sustenance could be withheld if the attending physician in consultation with next-of-kin or legally appointed representative, felt that sustenance would make the patient uncomfortable or would not improve their condition.

Further reading:
Onwuteaka Philipsen, B.D. et al (2003) Euthanasia and other end-of-life decisions in the Netherlands in 1990, 1995 and 2001. *Lancet* 361(9381) 395-9

House of Lords (2004) *Assisted Dying for the Terminally Ill Bill.* London: The Stationery Office

Summary: this would provide for help with suicide for an adult who is terminally ill and whose suffering is unbearable. The procedure would involve the patient signing a declaration which could be revoked at any time and which is to be witnessed and signed by two independent people one of whom must be a solicitor and neither of whom can be either of the physicians or a family member or an employee of the health care establishment. It outlines the duties of both attending and consultant physicians who must be sure in their diagnosis and sure to offer palliative/hospice care and/or pain control. The Bill would also provide for conscientious objection by the physician, and for insurance, psychiatric referral, monitoring and documentation and a terminally ill patient's right to ask for symptom relief.

Further reading:
Royal College of General Practitioners and Royal College of Physicians (2001) Medical treatment at the end of life: a position statement. *Clinical Medicine* 1(2) 115-117

Human Genetics Commission (2004) *Choosing the future: genetics and reproductive decision making.* London: HGC

Summary: whilst progress in genetics means we can identify genetic disorders and reduce the risk of our children having them, there are worries about what the long-term effect of this understanding will have on our society and what value we place on human life. The document looks at progress in genetics and reproduction, prenatal screening, diagnostic and genetics services and possible future developments. It goes on to look at some of the arguments surrounding:

- prenatal testing and the decisions to be made when an abnormality is found
- the feasibility of screening whole populations for certain rare diseases
- treatments to make pregnancy viable for menopausal women and conception possible for subfertile/infertile men
- treatments in utero or in vitro for identified genetic disorders
- embryo selection: choosing an embryo without a disorder to prevent a baby being born with a condition or to treat a sibling who has the condition

This document is part of a consultation process. At the end of 2005 the Commission will report their findings to the Government.

Further reading:
Aspis, S. (2001) Disability and the 1967 Abortion Act. *RCM Midwives Journal* 4(10) 338

Lewis, M. (2003) Is abortion due to handicap ethical? *British Journal of Midwifery* 11(7) 442-4

House of Commons (2004) *Mental Capacity Bill.* London: The Stationery Office

Summary: this would update and reform the law in cases where decisions are made on behalf of people who cannot make decisions for themselves. These are adults who are born incapacitated or who have lost mental capacity as the result of dementia or brain injury, defined according to a set of key principles. The decisions concern personal welfare, finance, business etc. The Bill would provide for:

- new rules to govern research involving people with mental incapacity
- rules to govern advance decisions to refuse treatment i.e. Living wills
- appointing an Independent Consultant to give advice about certain decisions
- making neglect or ill treatment a criminal offence
- a new Court of Protection employing a Public Guardian

Human Tissue Act 2004: chapter 30. London: The Stationery Office

Summary: in his report *The removal, retention and use of human organs and tissue from post mortem examination (2001,* see above) the Chief Medical Officer recommended a revision of the law following concerns raised in the Kennedy (2001), Redfern (2001) and Isaacs (2003) reports in which the crucial issue was the taking and holding of human material without consent. The Act replaces the *Human Tissue Act 1961*, the *Anatomy Act 1984* and the *Human Organs Transplant Act 1989* (see above). The Act is divided into 3 parts:

1. deals with consent for the use of organs taken from deceased bodies; the penalties for not obtaining consent; what to do with human material taken before the Act comes into force; and the limited circumstances where human material from living persons may be stored and used without consent. It does not cover the removal of organs from living persons

2. provides for a Human Tissue Authority - it prohibits any of the above activity without a licence issued by the Authority which must to draw up and circulate codes of practice and regulate transplants between living persons. The Act also provides for inspectorates of anatomy and pathology and of organs and tissues for human use

3. the Act allows hospitals to preserve organs whilst seeking consent for transplant; provides for the disposal of human material; prohibits the use of human material for DNA analysis (with certain exceptions) and allows museums to transfer or dispose of human remains

Further reading:

Department of Health (2003) *Investigation of events that followed the death of Cyril Mark Isaacs.* London: The Stationery Office

Samanta, A. et al (2004) Who owns my body - thee or me? The human tissue story continues. *Clinical Medicine* 4(4) 327-331

Supplementary Reading

Audit Commission (2000) *The journey to race equality: delivering improved services to local communities.* London: Audit Commission

Data Protection Act 1984: chapter 35. London: HMSO

Department of Health (2000) *An inquiry into quality and practice within the NHS arising from the actions of Rodney Ledward: the report.* (chair Jean Ritchie) London: Department of Health

Employment Rights Act 1996: chapter 18. London: The Stationery Office

Home Office and Department of Health (2000) *No secrets: guidance on developing and implementing multi-agency policies and procedures to protect vulnerable adults from abuse.* London: Department of Health

House of Lords (2002) *Stem cell research.* London: The Stationery Office

Nursing and Midwifery Council (2001) *Covert administration of medicines.* London: NMC

Office for National Statistics (annual) *Abortion statistics: legal abortions carried under the 1967 Abortion Act in England and Wales.* London: The Stationery Office

New, B. and Neuberger, J. (2002) *Hidden assets: values and decision-making in the NHS.* London: King's Fund

Royal College of Paediatrics and Child Health (1997) *Withholding or withdrawing life saving treatment in children.* (chair Neil McIntosh) London: Royal College of Paediatrics and Child Health

Staley, Kristina (2001) *Voices, values and health: involving the public in moral decisions.* London: King's Fund

Weissbrodt, D. and Anti-Slavery International (2002) *Abolishing slavery and its contemporary forms.* New York: United Nations

Applying for Jobs

Suggested Reading

Banks, C. (2003) How to interview effectively. *Nursing Times* 99(35) 52-3

BMJ Classified (1996) *Career focus: information that helps develop careers.* London: BMJ Publishing Group

Chambers, R. et al (2000) *Opportunities and options in medical careers.* Abingdon: Radcliffe Medical Press

Davison, N. (2004) Securing your first job. *Nursing Times* 100(19) 44-5

Freeman, A. E. L. and Wozniak, E. R. (2001) Preparing for consultant interview: advice from a regional advisor. *Current Paediatrics* 11(6) 470-4

Hoban, V. (2003) How to write a CV. *Nursing Times* 99(27) 52-3

Howard, S. (1999) *Creating a successful CV.* London: Dorling Kindersley

Little Tim (1996) *Power CVs and interview letters that really work.* Richmond: Langley Publishing

MacCallum, E. (2001) The first step to finding your first job. *Mental Health Practice* 4(6) 30-1

McKenzie, S. (2001) Writing your curriculum vitae. *Hospital Medicine* 62(9) 568-70

Marino, K. (2000) *Resumes for the healthcare professional.-2e* Chichester: John Wiley

Mumford, C.J. (2000) *Medical job interview: secrets for success.* Oxford: Blackwell

Robotham, M. (2001) How to make yourself just the job. *Nursing Times* 97(22) 24-5

Robotham, M. (2001) How to shine at the interview. *Nursing Times* 97(22) 26-7

Organisations

BRITISH ASSOCIATION OF SOCIAL WORKERS

16 Kent St, BIRMINGHAM B5 6RD

☎ 0121 622 3911

www.basw.co.uk

PURPOSE: "...the largest association representing social work and social workers in the UK....here to help, support, advise and campaign...."

BRITISH MEDICAL ASSOCIATION

BMA House, Tavistock Square, LONDON WC1H 9JP

☎ 020 7387 4499

www.bma.org.uk

PURPOSE: "We put the profession's democratically reached views to national administrations and many other influential bodies. We are an independent trade union officially recognised by government and the pay review bodies for negotiation on doctors' pay and conditions."

COMMUNITY AND DISTRICT NURSING ASSOCIATION

Walpole House, 18-22 Bond Street, Ealing LONDON W5 5AA

☎ 020 8231 0180

www.cdna.tvu.ac.uk

PURPOSE: "...to provide a quality industrial relations and professional service...and to lead and influence policy making decisions on professional issues relating to health care in the community...."

COMMUNITY PRACTITIONER & HEALTH VISITORS' ASSOCIATION
(was Health Visitors' Association)

40 Bermondsey Street, London, SE1 3UD

☎ 020 7939 7000

www.msf.org.uk/cphva.html

PURPOSE: "a professional organisation (and trade union)...for all nurse members in the primary health care team...with a strong focus on health promotion, preventive health care and the broad issues around public health."

DEPARTMENT OF HEALTH

Richmond House, 79 Whitehall, London, SW1A 2NS

☎ 020 7210 4850 (for general enquiries: open 9am - 5pm)

www.dh.gov.uk

DEPARTMENT FOR WORK AND PENSIONS (was Dept of Social Security)

Correspondence Unit, Room 540, The Adelphi, 1-11 John Adam St, LONDON WC2N 6HT

☎ 020 7712 2171

www.dss.gov.uk

GENERAL MEDICAL COUNCIL

Regent's Place, 350 Euston Road, LONDON NW1 3JN

☎ 020 7580 7642

www.gmc-uk.org

PURPOSE: " a charity... whose purpose is the protection, promotion and maintenance of the health and safety of the community. We have strong and effective legal powers designed to maintain the standards the public have the right to expect of doctors. We are not here to protect the medical profession...Our job is to protect patients."

GENERAL SOCIAL CARE COUNCIL

Goldings House, 2 Hay's Lane, LONDON SE1 2HB

☎ 020 7397 5100

www.gscc.org.uk/

PURPOSE: established in October 2001, the GSCC regulates social care workers. It sets codes of conduct and practice; regulates social work education and training and establishes a register of social care workers.

HEALTH PROFESSIONS COUNCIL

Park House, 184 Kennington Park Road, LONDON SE11 4BU

☎ 0845 3573 456

www.hpc-uk.org

PURPOSE: the HPC replaces the Council for Professions Supplementary to Medicine. It has been set up to regulate 12 healthcare professions - such as chiropodists, speech therapists, physiotherapists etc - with a view to safeguarding the health and wellbeing of patients and ensuring the professions are qualified and competent.

INDEPENDENT MIDWIVES ASSOCIATION

1 The Great Quarry, GUILDFORD GU1 3XN

☎ 01483 821104

www.independentmidwives.org.uk

PURPOSE: "Independent Midwives are fully qualified midwives who, in order to practice the midwife's role to its fullest extent, have chosen to work outside the NHS in a self employed capacity, although we support its aims and ideals. The midwife's role encompasses the care of women during pregnancy, birth and afterwards."

JOSEPH ROWNTREE FOUNDATION

The Homestead, 40 Water End, YORK YO30 6WP

☎ 01904 629241

www.jrf.org.uk

PURPOSE: an independent social policy research and development charity; supports a wide programme of research and development projects in housing, social care and social policy.

KING'S FUND

11-13 Cavendish Square, London W1G 0AN

☎ 020 7307 2400

www.kingsfund.org.uk

PURPOSE: "... to stimulate and disseminate good practice and innovation in health and related services....make an independent and influential, contribution to the development of health policy nationally and internationally."

NATIONAL INSTITUTE FOR SOCIAL WORK

5 Tavistock Place, LONDON WC1H 9SN

☎ 020 7387 9681

www.nisw.org.uk

PURPOSE: established in 1961, the Institute provides staff training, research and specialist library resources for the personal social services, "...actively raising standards and promoting good practice in the public, independent and voluntary sectors".

NURSING AND MIDWIFERY COUNCIL

23 Portland Place, LONDON W1B 1PZ

☎ 020 7637 7181

www.nmc-uk.org

PURPOSE: the NMC regulates nursing, midwifery and health visiting. It maintains a register of nurses midwives and health visitors, sets standards for their education, practice and conduct, provides advice and considers allegations of misconduct or unfitness to practice.

THE QUEEN'S NURSING INSTITUTE

3 Albemarle Way, London, EC1V 4RQ

☎ 020 7490 4227

www.qni.org.uk

PURPOSE: "... promotes the highest standards of nursing in the community... to encourage the best possible community health care and public health"

ROYAL COLLEGE OF MIDWIVES - RCM

15 Mansfield Street, London, W1G 9NH

☎ 020 7312 3535

www.rcm.org.uk

PURPOSE: "...exists to protect and advance the interests of midwives/midwifery...supplying professional/educational services...industrial relations advice, support and information"

ROYAL COLLEGE OF NURSING - RCN

20 Cavendish Square, London, W1G 0RN

☎ 0845 772 6100

www.rcn.org.uk

PURPOSE: a trade union that serves its 303,000+ members in professional matters, labour relations and education.

WORLD HEALTH ORGANIZATION

Avenue Appia 20, 1211 GENEVA 27, Switzerland

☎ 004122 791 2111

www.who.int

Abbreviations

ASC	Action for Sick Children
CHAI	Commission for Healthcare Audit and Inspection
CHI	Commission for Health Improvement
DHA	district health authority
DHSS	Department of Health and Social Security
DOH	Department of Health
DSS	Department of Social Security
ENB	English National Board
FHSA	family health service authority
GP	general practitioner
IV	intra venous
NAWCH	National Association for the Welfare of Children in Hospital (now ASC)
NHSE	National Health Service Executive
NHSME	National Health Service Management Executive
NICE	National Institute for Clinical Excellence
NSF	National Service Framework
PCG / PCT	primary care group / trust
PREP	post-registration education and practice
R&D	research and development
RCM	Royal College of Midwifery
RCN	Royal College of Nursing
RHA	regional health authority
UKCC	United Kingdom Central Council for Nursing Midwifery & Health Visiting
WHO	World Health Organisation

Websites

Audit Commission	www.audit-commission.gov.uk
BMA	www.bma.org.uk
CCTA Government Information Service	www.open.gov.uk
Commission for Healthcare Audit and Inspection	www.chai.org.uk
Commission for Social Care Inspection	www.csci.org.uk
Department of Health	www.dh.gov.uk
Department of Social Security	www.dss.gov.uk
Electronic Library for Social Care	www.elsc.org.uk
General Medical Council	www.gmc-uk.org
General Social Care Council	www.gscc.org.uk
Health Professions Council	www.hpc-uk.org
King's Fund	www.kingsfund.org.uk/
MIDIRS	www.midirs.org.uk
National Electronic Library for Health	www.nelh.nhs.uk
National Institute for Social Work	www.nisw.org.uk
National Library for Health	www.library.nhs.uk
Nursing and Midwifery Council	www.nmc-uk.org
NMAP	www.nmap.ac.uk
Official Publications	www.official-documents.co.uk
OMNI (medical gateway)	www.omni.ac.uk
Royal College of Midwives	www.rcm.org.uk
Royal College of Nursing	www.rcn.org.uk
Sainsbury Centre for Mental Health	www.scmh.org.uk
SCHARR	www.shef.ac.uk/uni/academic/R-Z/scharr
SOSIG (social science gateway)	www.sosig.ac.uk
WHO	www.who.int/en/

Alphabetical Index